Is It a Choice?

Answers to the Most Frequently Asked Questions About Gay and Lesbian People

ERIC MARCUS

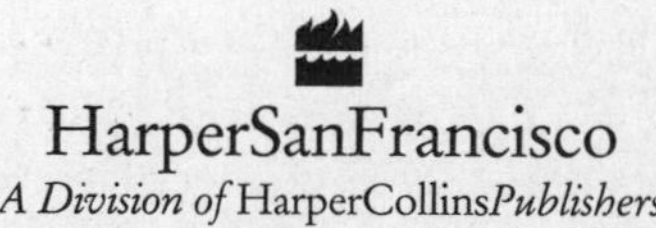

HarperSanFrancisco
A Division of HarperCollins*Publishers*

Also by Eric Marcus

Pessimisms
Making Gay History
What If Someone I Know Is Gay?
Together Forever
Icebreaker, with Rudy Galindo
Why Suicide?
Breaking the Surface, with Greg Louganis
Making History
The Male Couple's Guide

Please visit my Web site: www.ericmarcus.com

HarperCollins books may be purchased for educational, business, or sales promotional use. For information please write: Special Markets Department, HarperCollins Publishers, 10 East 53rd Street, New York, NY 10022.

HarperCollins Web site: http://www.harpercollins.com

THIRD EDITION
FIRST HARPER SAN FRANCISCO EDITION PUBLISHED IN 1993

Library of Congress Cataloging-in-Publication Data is available.

ISBN-13: 978–0–06–083280–3
ISBN-10: 0–06–083280–0

06 07 08 09 RRD(H) 10 9 8 7 6 5 4 3 2

For Ryan & Evan

Contents

Acknowledgments

Many thanks to my original editor, Barbara Moulton, for sharing my enthusiasm for *Is It a Choice?* at a time when nearly no one else did; to Alison Ames, for generously providing a very comfortable place to work; to Barry Owen, for his help with the proposal; and to Ann Northrop, for her wisdom, encouragement, and support.

Special thanks to all those who suggested questions, offered sage advice, and/or read the manuscript, including Lisa Bach, Dr. Betty Berzon, Mark Burstein, Cate Corcoran, Christine Egan, Ilan Greenberg, Cynthia Grossman, Fred Hertz's grandmother, Alex Lash, Aaron Levaco, Peggy Levine, Matthew Lore, Cecilia Marcus (my mom), May Marcus (my grandmother), Steven Mazzola, Bill Megevick, Judy Montague, Jessica Morris, Joel Roselin, Phil Roselin, Bill Russell, Stuart Schear, Bill Smith, Scott Terranella, and Nick Wingfield.

For the second edition, many thanks to my editor, Liz Perle, and her eagle-eyed assistant David Hennessy, for their unwavering support and help. Thank you also to my researchers, Jennifer Finlay and Stephen Milioti. Thank you, Nancy Kokolj, for reviewing the finished manuscript. And a special thank you to my meticulous copy editor, Carl Walesa.

For the third edition, thank you to my agent, Joy Harris, my editor Gideon Weil, Carl Walesa (again), and the many people from around the world who contributed new questions and offered their suggestions. A special thanks to Ryan Marcus, my nephew, who made certain that this latest edition is anchored in the twenty-first century. Thank you again to Stephen Milioti for making certain my answers were grounded in fact; and thank you, as well, to Don Press and Bronwen Pardes. And, as always, to my partner in life, Barney M. Karpfinger, thank you for so much.

Introduction

Not long ago, while on a flight from my home in New York City to New Orleans, the woman seated to my right asked me a couple of seemingly innocent questions: "Are you traveling on business?" and "What kind of work do you do?" I'd learned from past experience that answering innocent questions can easily lead to uncomfortably long silences, which are especially uncomfortable when you're seated elbow-to-elbow in a steel tube at forty thousand feet.

I remember one fellow, an Israeli, who started a conversation with me just as our plane left the ground on the way from New York to Los Angeles. A few questions later, after he learned that I wrote books about gay people, the conversation ended. My seatmate never said another word during the six-hour flight, and upon our landing in L.A. he was out of his seat before we reached the gate.

Like everyone else, I'm human, so I try to avoid uncomfortable situations. And I had an uneasy feeling on the New Orleans–bound flight that the woman asking the questions might not welcome the gay man seated next to her. I'd already overheard a piece of a conversation she'd had with a colleague across the aisle about an article in *USA Today* that had something to do with gay people. And from the tone of the conversation, I thought I had reason to be wary.

Her questions and answers followed a predictable progression: "Oh, you're a writer. What do you write?" "I write books." "What kinds of books?" "Nonfiction." "What kinds of nonfiction?"

I wasn't trying to be coy, but I was hoping that my less than expansive answers would get me off the hook. My seatmate was undaunted, and sure enough, after I told her that most of my books were about gay people, there was silence. But not for long, because then Lillian started telling me about her youngest son, of whom she was very proud. He wasn't like his other brothers, who were athletic, but instead loved to sing and dance and was always the star of his school plays. She pulled his school photo from her purse, showed it to me, and promptly burst into tears.

"I think my son is gay," Lillian said, "and I don't know what to do." She explained that she had never talked to anyone about her concerns besides her husband. Ten-year-old Andrew was already getting called names at elementary school, and she feared for his safety. She loved her son and wanted to do everything she could to make certain he'd grow up to be a well-adjusted gay kid. For a moment *I* was speechless, and then I had a few questions of my own. (For more about Andrew and his mom, have a look at chapter 5, "For Parents of Gay Children.")

I've been answering questions about homosexuality for what feels like a very long time—beginning in 1976, to be exact. But it wasn't until 1988, when my first book—*The Male Couple's Guide*—was published, that I realized just how little most people knew about homosexuality.

My publisher sent me on a ten-day publicity trip across the United States, during which time I discovered that no one was interested in the substance of my book. All the questions that came my way were very basic: "How do you know you're a homosexual?" "How do parents react to a gay child?" "Why do gay people want to get married?"

Still, it wasn't until I discovered that my own friends had the same basic questions everyone else had that I realized there was a desperate need for a book that offered clear, concise answers about gay and lesbian people and the lives we lead.

Shortly after returning home from my cross-country trip, I had dinner with my good friends Duffie and Simeon. She's a journalist, and he's a lawyer. Recently married. Highly educated. New York sophisticates. I thought nothing of complaining to them about my experiences on the road: "You can't *believe* the stupid questions I have to answer." Duffie asked, "What kinds of stupid questions?" I rattled off a long list, including the one question I was asked most often: "Is it a choice?"

Duffie turned bright red, paused, and said, "Those don't sound like stupid questions to me." Simeon said: "It's *not* a choice?" I almost fell off my chair. They were my friends! They had known me for years! They lived in Manhattan, for God's sake! But they didn't know. After thinking about it for a little while, I realized that Duffie and I, after our initial discussion when we met in graduate school, had never talked about the fact that I was gay. I had just assumed that Duffie and Simeon knew about gay people. But they didn't.

The next week, I had dinner with friends of mine and theirs. Kate and Rick are a little older than Duffie and Simeon. Totally cool people. Kate's a potter, and Rick is a brilliant economist. I assumed they'd be as shocked as I was at how little Duffie and Simeon knew. Well, you can easily imagine how the rest of the conversation played out. Kate and Rick were surprised by my surprise and suggested that I was mistaken in my assumptions. No kidding.

After that night with Kate and Rick, I was determined to write a book that included all the questions I had ever been asked and then some. You're holding in your hands the third edition of the original *Is It a Choice?*, which over the years has been translated into Spanish, Hebrew, Polish, Thai, and Japanese. So now the questions come to me via e-mail from as far away as Bangladesh, Jordan, and Nepal.

The questions and answers you'll find in *Is It a Choice?* come from many different sources. Most of the questions are my own; others were gathered from friends, family, people I've met through my travels; and still others have come from readers around the world. For the answers to the many questions I've included here, I talked to lots of people, including experts from a variety of fields. I've also drawn information from magazine and newspaper articles, as well as scores of books and Web sites. And I've read reports and studies, lots of them.

As you'll see, my responses range from exceedingly brief to detailed and involved. You'll find plenty of anecdotes, opinions, and conjecture, but some of the answers will leave you with even more questions, because some of the questions I've included don't yet have definitive answers.

The answers I offer in *Is It a Choice?* are mostly *my* answers, which means they're not the only possible answers to the questions I pose. Other gay and lesbian people would likely answer these questions differently, because gay men and women are a diverse population with different values and different ways of looking at our world.

Some of you may be disappointed to discover in the answers I offer that gay people aren't nearly as exotic as we're sometimes portrayed, especially by those individuals and organizations that would have you believe we are forever parading, scantily clad in black leather or sequins, down the main streets of cities near and far.

In fact, some gay and lesbian people *are* pretty exotic and dress up in very imaginative ways, but the same can be said of some heterosexual people. (Have you ever been to Mardi Gras or Carnival?) But in writing *Is It a Choice*? I've chosen to stick pretty close to the broad middle of lesbian and gay life. And I've also limited myself primarily to addressing questions about the "L" and "G" of the LGBT acronym often used to denote the lesbian, gay, bisexual, and transgender communities.

You'll meet all kinds of people in *Is It a Choice?* Some give answers to questions; others provide stories that help support a point. When I've used quotes or anecdotes from experts and public people, such as gay and lesbian rights advocates, I've used complete names. When I quote private citizens or use their anecdotes—some of which are composites drawn from several people—I've used only first names and changed identifying details for reasons of privacy.

Not all the possible questions about homosexuality are included in this relatively brief volume, nor are all the answers. If there's a question I've missed that you would like answered, or if you have an answer to a question that I failed to answer adequately, contact me through my Web site: www.ericmarcus.com.

And remember, there really is no such thing as a stupid question—except for the question you don't ask.

1

The Basics

? What is a homosexual?

A homosexual is a person whose feelings of sexual attraction are for someone of the same gender: male for male, female for female. In contrast, a heterosexual is a person whose feelings of attraction are for someone of the opposite gender.

The word *homosexual* was first used by Karl Maria Kertbeny in an 1869 pamphlet in which he argued for the repeal of Prussia's antihomosexual laws. (Prussia is now part of northern Germany.) *Homosexual* combines the Greek word for "same" with the Latin word for "sex."

Homosexual people come in all shapes and sizes and from all walks of life, just like heterosexual people do, and are part of every community and every family. This means that everyone knows someone who is homosexual. Most people just don't realize that they know, and perhaps love, someone who is homosexual, because many—if not most—homosexual people keep their sexual orientation a secret.

I wish I had known what a homosexual was when I was growing up in the 1960s and 1970s in Kew Gardens, New York, a comparatively bucolic New York City neighborhood about forty-five minutes from Manhattan by subway. At first I didn't know exactly what a homosexual was, except that homosexuals were something very bad and disgusting. The popular image for someone of my generation was a creepy-looking guy in an overcoat who hid behind bushes and tried to lure children into his clutches with candy.

As I grew into adolescence, I still wasn't exactly sure what a homosexual was, never having seen one on television or having met one, but I knew that the most horrible thing you could call someone was a "faggot." In summer camp there was always at least one boy who got tagged with that label. It was usually someone who always struck out at baseball. He was despised by the other boys and shunned by the girls.

One summer, when I was fourteen, I was that boy. It was also around this time when I was just beginning to understand that "faggot" meant more than just being bad at baseball. It had to do with not being like other boys, who at that age were starting to get girl-crazy in a way that made no sense to me. I can't say I had any memorable attraction to those of my own gender back then, but I do recall thinking that my strapping eighteen-year-old counselor, Ted, was kind of cute—an observation I knew not to share with my bunkmates.

I was sixteen years old when I finally met someone I knew to be homosexual, and I was both shocked and relieved. Bob was no creepy-looking guy in an overcoat. He was a smart, devastatingly handsome (to me), and very confident college student who lived down the block. He didn't lurk behind shrubs, and he never once offered me candy. He did, however, help dispel all the myths I'd grown up with about homosexuality.

Bob was the first person to explain to me that a homosexual is simply a man or woman whose feelings of sexual attraction are for someone of the same gender. One man could meet and fall in love with another man, my new friend explained, and one woman could fall in love with another woman. So simple, but to me it was a revolutionary idea, and it changed my life, especially since I had a wild crush on Bob and could now do what any normal sixteen-year-old would do: imagine a life that included living happily ever after with the object of my affections.

? What is a gay person? Why do gay people call themselves "gay"?

A gay person is a man or woman who is a homosexual. *Gay* is a synonym for *homosexual.* The word has been used publicly by gay people since the late 1960s, when *gay* was adopted by homosexual men and women in the early gay civil rights movement and incorporated into slogans like "Gay is good!" *Gay* was seen as a positive alternative to the clinical-sounding *homosexual.*

Gay was used as slang in place of *homosexual* as far back as the 1920s, almost exclusively within the homosexual community. If, for example, you wanted to indicate to a friend that a club or bar you planned to go to was frequented by homosexuals, you would say that it was a "gay place" or that there was a "gay crowd."

One of the early examples of *gay* being used in print to mean "homosexual" occurred in 1947. Lisa Ben, a young Hollywood secretary, used the word as part of the subtitle for a newsletter for lesbians that she published on her office typewriter. Lisa called her newsletter *Vice Versa: America's Gayest Magazine.* Other homosexual people knew that Lisa didn't mean her magazine was simply full of fun, which is what most people at the time would have thought, because *gay* was a word then typically used to mean "happy" or "fun," as in "We had such a gay time at the party."

Not all homosexual people like using the word *gay* to describe themselves. And since *gay* has come to be used most often in association with male homosexuals, many homosexual women prefer to be called *lesbians.* (See "What do gay people like to be called?" at the end of this chapter.)

? What is a lesbian?

A lesbian is a woman whose primary feelings of sexual attraction are for other women. In other words, a lesbian is a homosexual woman. Like gay men, lesbians come in all shapes and sizes and from all walks of life.

The word *lesbian* derives from the name of a Greek island, Lesbos, where Sappho, a teacher known for her poetry celebrating love between women, established a school for young women in the sixth century BC. Over time, the word *lesbian,* which once simply meant someone who lived on Lesbos, came to mean a woman who, like Sappho and her followers, loved other women.

? Do gay men find all men sexually attractive? Do lesbians find all women sexually attractive?

No. Like most heterosexuals, gay people are pretty picky about the kind of person they find sexually attractive. So for all the heterosexual guys out there who are afraid that the gay guy at the gym or in their school shower is looking at them because they want to have sex with them, it's okay to relax. They're probably looking at you because gay people, like all humans, are generally curious and like to look at other humans, clothed or unclothed.

What is a bisexual?

Bisexual is the term used to describe a person who has feelings of sexual attraction for both men and women. But I think the term is misleading, because it suggests that such a person has the same strength of feelings for both men and women. Humans are far more complicated than that and more typically have stronger feelings of sexual attraction for one gender than the other.

It was Alfred Kinsey who, in his landmark studies in the 1940s and 1950s on male and female sexuality, first revealed the rich variety of sexual feelings and expression. He developed a seven-point rating scale to represent human sexual attraction and experience.

The Kinsey scale has a range of zero to six. The zero category includes all people who are exclusively heterosexual in their feelings of sexual attraction and report no homosexual experience or attraction. Category six includes those who are exclusively homosexual in experience and attraction. Everyone else falls somewhere in between.

Some people are under the mistaken impression that people who are bisexual are involved in sexual relationships with both men and women at the same time. Though this may be the case for some people, most women and men who identify as bisexual and are in couple relationships have only a single partner at a time.

Are bisexuals just gay people who are afraid to admit they're gay?

No. Most men and women who identify as bisexual are indeed bisexual. If there's some confusion about this, it's because some homosexuals, as they come to terms with accepting themselves, may at first say that they are bisexual, even thought they're not. That's what I did.

In my last year of high school I confided to a close male friend—who I thought might be gay—that I was bisexual. By this time I already knew I was gay because of the crush I had on Bob, the college student down the block, and I wasn't the least bit interested in having a physical relationship with a woman. But somehow, "bisexual" didn't sound nearly as bad as "gay," and I really wasn't ready to acknowledge to myself or the world the truth about my feelings. I was, needless to say, a fairly tortured and somewhat confused adolescent.

I figured if I said that I was bisexual, then in the eyes of the world—and in my own eyes—I was at least half heterosexual. I rationalized that I could keep one foot in the gay world and the other safely in the heterosexual world, in word if not in deed. And I imagined that people would have an easier time accepting me if they thought I "went both ways." But within a couple of years, when I felt more comfortable about being gay, I gave up claiming I was bisexual.

Unfortunately, because of gay people like me, many people have the misconception that all men and women who say they are bisexual are homosexuals who are afraid to admit the truth about themselves. This is simply a misconception. Yes, some people who claim to be bisexual, as I did, are gay, but there are many people who have feelings of sexual attraction, to varying degrees, for both men and women—and they are called "bisexuals."

Is bisexuality the same as living "on the down low"?

No. "On the down low," or "on the DL," is a slang term that originated among African Americans. It is used to refer to men in heterosexual relationships who also have sex with men. Most often these men do not consider themselves to be gay or bisexual, and, in general, they keep this aspect of their sexual lives secret from their female partners and their families. They're in hiding, or, in other words, "on the down low."

What makes this a little confusing is that men who live on the down low are engaging in bisexual behavior and have a homosexual or bisexual sexual orientation. But they generally think of themselves as heterosexual men who have sex with men. If it sounds like I'm describing a person who is a mental contortionist, you're right. But however confusing it may seem, this is simply another way that some men have chosen to adapt to living in communities that are less than accepting of people who live an openly gay life.

Unfortunately, life on the down low usually involves unsuspecting female partners who are likely to have no idea that the men they are partnered with are leading secret lives.

For a fictional look into the lives of men who live on the down low, a great place to start is with the best-selling novels of E. Lynn Harris.

What is a transsexual or transgendered person?

The words *transsexual* and *transgendered* are moving targets, and it seems that no two people I've spoken with can agree on exactly what they mean. So I turned for help to someone who works with transgendered and transsexual youth at a group home in New York City. What follows is a paraphrase of what he told me.

Transgender is an umbrella term that covers a broad range of "gender expression," including drag queens and kings (see chapter 18, "Miscellaneous Questions"), cross-dressers, transgenderists, and transsexuals. These individuals are often people who find their gender identity—their sense of themselves as male or female—in conflict with their anatomical gender.

Transsexuals are people who have a gender-identity conflict. Some, although not all, transsexuals feel as though they are trapped in the wrong body. In other words, a man may feel he belongs in a woman's body. And a woman may feel she belongs in a man's body.

Some transsexuals may live part-time in their self-defined gender, dressing and behaving in a manner generally associated with that gender. Others choose to live full-time in their self-identified gender. Some transsexuals also choose to undergo sexual-reassignment surgery so their anatomical gender matches their self-identified gender.

? Is that the same as a transvestite or drag queen?

See chapter 18, "Miscellaneous Questions."

? How can you tell who is gay? What do gay men and lesbians look like? Why are gay men effeminate and lesbians masculine?

For the most part, you can't tell who is gay or lesbian from appearances, unless the man or woman in question is wearing a button or symbol that explicitly identifies him or her as homosexual.

Years ago the common assumption was that all gay and lesbian people were easily identifiable by well-established stereotypical mannerisms, affectations, dress, and so on. The typical lesbian was masculine in appearance and behavior and dressed in mannish clothing. The typical gay man was effeminate and paid more attention to the way he dressed and his grooming than "normal" guys. He might even wear a little makeup.

It turns out that many effeminate men—but certainly not all—are gay and that many masculine women—but certainly not all—are lesbians. But by and large, gay and lesbian people, like heterosexual people, come in all shapes, sizes, colors, and ages, as well as degrees of masculinity and femininity. And you certainly don't have to be a gay man or heterosexual woman to enjoy a good pedicure or facial every now and then.

? Do gay people choose to be gay? Are you born gay? Is it inherited? Can your parents make you gay? Can you be seduced or recruited into being gay? Do you become gay because of a bad sexual experience or because of sexual abuse?

We all make choices about how we conduct our lives. But there are fundamental aspects of ourselves about which we don't get a choice—eye color, fingerprints, and left- or right-handedness, for example. We also don't get a choice about our feelings of sexual attraction. I didn't choose my same-gender feelings of sexual attraction any more than my brother and sister chose their opposite-gender feelings of sexual attraction.

From an early age my younger brother thought women's breasts were the most wondrous creations on earth. In stark contrast, I had no idea what all the excitement was about. But Greg Louganis, the Olympic diver—now, *that* was a different story. Seeing Greg on the diving board at the 1984 Olympics made me think *he* was the most wondrous creation on earth.

No one knows exactly how feelings of sexual attraction get bestowed on each of us or how early in life, although contemporary research strongly suggests that there are both a genetic and a biological basis for what is proving to be an exceedingly complex puzzle. But whatever your own personal beliefs about how we come into existence—Darwin, God, and/or Mother Nature—your feelings of sexual attraction come to you very early in life (before or after birth) and are yours and yours alone and remain yours until the day you die—just like your fingerprints, your eye color, and your right- or left-handedness. And like these other genetically inheritable traits, sexual orientation has a genetically inheritable component—but no one knows exactly to what degree it is inheritable or what the mechanics of that inheritance might be. Like so much about us humans, sexual orientation remains something of a mystery.

So whether some quack psychoanalyst would like to attribute homosexuality to domineering mothers or passive fathers, whether parents try to pin the blame on a bad sexual experience their child may have had, or whether your best friend thinks you're a lesbian only because you were seduced by your college roommate, look at your fingerprints and remind yourself that feelings of sexual attraction are innate, immutable, and uniquely your own. What we choose to do about those feelings is an entirely different matter, which I address in the next question.

One final thought on this subject: if all the women who have had bad sexual experiences with men became lesbians, I suspect there wouldn't be very many heterosexual women left. Think about that.

Can gay people choose to be heterosexual if they really want to be?

Well, yes, sort of, at least when it comes to behavior. And heterosexuals can be gay if they want to be as well, at least when it comes to *their* behavior; they may not like having sex with someone of the same gender, but they can certainly do it.

But behaving heterosexually will not make a gay person's feelings of same-gender attraction go away, just as behaving homosexually will not make a heterosexual person's feelings of opposite-gender attraction go away. And, I might add, prayer won't make feelings of sexual attraction go away, either, despite what various religious leaders have claimed in the past and to this day. Nor will "conversion" programs that claim to make gay people straight change anyone's innate feelings.

Prayer and conversion programs may help individuals suppress their feelings of same-gender sexual attraction for a time, maybe even years, but those feelings remain, just waiting to reassert themselves. And, really, is expressing those feelings such a bad thing? After all, feelings of sexual attraction, when handled responsibly by consenting adults, don't hurt anyone, and have even been known to make people quite happy.

This is how I see it in personal terms: Just as my left-handed father was forced in the 1930s to learn to use his right hand adequately to perform all the functions that came naturally to his left hand, I could learn to do the things heterosexual men do, even though it doesn't come naturally to me. I don't think I would be all that good at it, I know it wouldn't be my first choice, and I also know that in a very short time I would feel frustrated and more than a little bit irritable, but no more or less so than a heterosexual who was forced to live as a homosexual.

Plenty of people with same-gender sexual orientation choose for all kinds of reasons not to express their feelings of attraction and consciously decide to live a heterosexual life. Are they happy about it? Well, yes and no, but mostly no, if you judge by the past twenty years' worth of conversations I've had with and e-mails I've received from men and women with same-gender orientation who were in heterosexual marriages—some for decades. These were generally people who felt torn between continuing in the outwardly heterosexual lives they'd created for themselves and, as one writer put it, "throwing myself from a cliff."

I know there are heterosexual people who believe that it shouldn't be any big deal for gay people to "go straight." But to them I offer this challenge: Try "going gay," and see how much you like it. And then imagine marrying a same-gender partner and living that way for the rest of your life. And don't forget the part about being monogamous. Then send me an e-mail in twenty years, and let me know how it worked out.

? If my parent or brother or sister is gay, does that mean I'll be gay, too?

We're back to genetics and biology. If your parent or sibling is gay, there may be a greater chance that you will be gay, too, than if your parent or sibling is not gay. Not because of association or influence, but because of genetics and biology. If there were reliable statistics about this that I felt comfortable with, I'd offer them. But there aren't.

I can tell you that in my family, as far as I know, I'm the only gay person to come along as far back as anyone can remember. (My grandmother remembers her great-grandmother, so we're talking mid-nineteenth century.) I have my suspicions about one great-uncle who was not the most masculine guy in the world, but as I said earlier in this chapter, not all effeminate men are gay.

? What about identical twins? If it's genetic, then if one is gay, the other must be, too, right?

This is where things get interesting. In a study of identical twins, the scientists Michael Bailey and Richard Pillard found that where one twin is gay, the other twin has an approximately 50 percent chance of being gay. If sexual orientation were strictly genetic, both identical twins would always be gay or always heterosexual. So there are clearly biological factors other than genetics at work here. Stay tuned.

? How do you know if you're gay?

The key to knowing your sexual orientation is recognizing your feelings of sexual attraction. The challenge for many gay and bisexual people is being honest with themselves about what they're feeling. Because society can be so unaccepting of them, it's difficult for many gay people to acknowledge and accept what they know in their heart of hearts to be true of themselves.

One of the big challenges I faced in college as I began telling friends that I was gay was explaining to them *how* I knew I was gay. Most often I answered their questions by asking them how they knew they were straight. They would usually answer that they had never thought about it or that they "just knew." Well, I just knew, too. For as long as I could remember I found certain men physically attractive, in the same way that I knew most men found certain women attractive and most women found certain men attractive.

Beyond that explanation, I usually tried to find an example my friends could relate to. One of the first people who asked me this question was my friend Cindy. The question came up during our junior year of college on a trip we made to New York City to see a ballet performance. I decided to use the ballet as an example of how I knew I was gay.

During intermission, I asked Cindy what she thought about the principal woman dancer. Cindy said that she thought she was an excellent performer and very beautiful. I told her that I felt exactly the same way.

Then I asked her what she thought of the virtually naked male dancer who had performed a masterful and aggressive solo just before intermission. I knew Cindy well enough to know what her answer would be. She said, as I expected, "Oh my God, he's so handsome! He's so sexy!" Again, I told her that I felt exactly the same way.

The handsome and sexy dancer had left us both a little breathless and filled with desire. Using that example, I was able to convey to my friend that the experience of being attracted to someone—a man, in this case—was little different for me than it was for her. It was an experience so automatic that we didn't have the chance to think about it before being hit by a quickening pulse. The difference, of course, was that almost everyone would consider Cindy's feelings for the dancer to be perfectly normal. And though my feelings felt perfectly normal to me, there are plenty of people who would choose a word other than *normal* to describe my response to the male dancer.

Do you have to have a sexual experience to know for sure?

No. Sexual orientation has everything to do with feelings of sexual attraction and nothing to do with actual experience. As you grow through childhood, you become aware of your feelings of attraction. That awareness, no matter your orientation, does not require actual physical experience. If you think back to your own early awareness of your attractions, more likely than not you knew whether you were attracted to members of the same gender, the opposite gender, or both long before becoming sexually active.

That said, a sexual experience can certainly help confirm what you already sense to be true. At least, that was my experience.

Are straight people ever attracted to someone of the same sex? Are gay people ever attracted to someone of the opposite sex?

Of course! Human sexuality is profoundly complex and not easily compartmentalized into the rigid categories we humans have created to try to bring some order to something that often defies order. So it should surprise no one that it's perfectly normal for a homosexual person to have feelings of sexual attraction for someone of the opposite gender, just as it's perfectly normal for a straight person to have feelings of sexual attraction for someone of the same gender. It doesn't mean that your feelings are strong enough to compel you to have sex with that person, but these feelings could easily be strong enough to make you feel good.

Even though these feelings of attraction are something almost all people experience at one time or another, they can still be very confusing. For example, the first time I had an erotic dream about a woman, I was probably twenty. I woke up in the morning stunned, wondering how I could possibly have had such a dream after finally accepting that I was gay. Could I have made a mistake? Was I really heterosexual?

Through the course of the day I realized that one heterosexual erotic dream was just that—nothing to get upset about. My feelings for men hadn't changed, and beyond that one dream—as well as a few others over the years—I had no strong feelings of sexual attraction for women.

After talking with friends about my dream, I discovered I wasn't the only gay man who had had a heterosexual erotic dream. And some of my straight friends acknowledged having had homosexual erotic dreams.

? If you have a homosexual experience, does that make you gay? If you have a heterosexual experience, does that make you straight?

No. Physical behavior doesn't determine or change your sexual orientation. Plenty of heterosexual people have had sexual relations with someone of the same gender, and plenty of gay and lesbian people have had sexual relations with someone of the opposite gender. These experiences have not changed anyone's basic sexual orientation, although they may have broadened a few horizons.

Is homosexuality normal? Is it unnatural?

I always hate when people answer a question with a question, but it seems appropriate here. What's normal? What's natural? And who gets to decide? To me, my sexual orientation seems quite normal and decidedly natural. Having sex with a woman felt abnormal and unnatural. Luckily for me, I found another man who feels the way I do and is as attracted to me as I am to him—in all kinds of ways—and we've been living what seems to me a pretty normal life as a couple for more than a decade.

So are we normal in the sense that we're in the majority? No. But neither are people who are left-handed or have blue eyes. Are we abnormal or unnatural because we don't conduct our sexual lives as God or nature intended? Well, what exactly did God and nature intend?

I've heard some people argue that God and nature determined that penile-vaginal intercourse is the only natural or normal way to be sexually active. If we accept this assumption, then heterosexuals who engage in sexual activity other than penile-vaginal intercourse are engaging in unnatural and abnormal acts. Welcome to the club!

Is homosexuality a mental illness?

No. But I think that some of the rabid bigots and antigay activists I've come across over the years have emotional problems.

For example, is it normal to place a telephone call to a radio talk show for the express purpose of telling the show's guest—me—that he deserves his rights, "including the right to be chained to my truck and dragged down the highway"? To me, that person sounds disturbed.

Gay people as a group were never mentally ill, but until 1973, when the American Psychiatric Association voted to remove homosexuality from its official list of mental illnesses, gay people had to live with the mental-illness label. (The American Psychological Association followed suit a little more than a year later.) The late psychologist Dr. Evelyn Hooker helped get the ball rolling in the mid-1950s when she demonstrated in a landmark study that gay men were on average just as sane as their nongay counterparts.

? Can homosexuality be cured? What methods have been tried?

Diseases can be cured. Sexual orientation is not a disease. Therefore, it can't be cured. In other words, you could no more "cure" a gay person of his or her feelings of sexual attraction than you could "cure" a heterosexual person of his or her feelings of sexual attraction.

But that hasn't prevented plenty of people, including licensed mental health professionals, from trying. And the methods they've used over the years are the kinds of things you might read about in a horror novel, including electroshock therapy, brain surgery, hormone injections, and even castration. Other methods used in the past have included aversion therapy, in which, for example, male homosexuals were shown erotic pictures of men at the same time that an electric shock was applied to their genitals or they were induced to vomit.

Although "curing" homosexuality is no longer the goal of mainstream mental health professionals, there are individuals and organizations that maintain programs to "help" gay people change their orientation, and some of these groups and individuals are alleged to employ a number of the now discredited methods.

I like what "Dear Abby," the advice columnist, has to say on this subject: "Any therapist who would take a gay person and try to change him or her should be in jail. What the psychiatrist should do is make the patient more comfortable with what he or she is—to be himself or herself." Amen!

? Are gay people more likely to molest children?

No. The most likely person to molest children is a heterosexual male. His most likely victim is a female child. For example, a study conducted by Children's Hospital in Denver found that between July 1, 1991, and June 30, 1992, only 1 percent of 387 cases of suspected child molestation involved a gay perpetrator. Overwhelmingly, the study found that boys and girls alike said they were abused by heterosexual male family members, including fathers, stepfathers, grandfathers, and uncles.

? What is the gay lifestyle?

There is no such thing as a "gay lifestyle," just as there is no such thing as a "heterosexual lifestyle." Gay and lesbian people, like all people, choose to live their lives in all different kinds of ways—or lifestyles—which may be very similar to yours or quite different.

Back in 1992, just after I moved back to New York City following the end of a long-term relationship, my friend Kate told me that she was worried that I'd go out and lead a wild "gay lifestyle." Based on her misconceptions, she feared that I would go out to gay clubs, dance all night, drink too much, take drugs, probably strip my shirt off when things got too hot, and maybe even have unprotected sex in a dark corner.

Of course, some gay men live a wild, urban, single lifestyle—as do some heterosexual men—but given what my friend knew about me and the life I had led in the past, I was more likely to be in bed, alone, at 10:00 p.m. than heading out the door for a wild night at the clubs.

? How many gay and lesbian people are there?

If you know, please write to me, because from what I know, no one really knows. I've read more than a few studies, none of which is definitive. Part of the problem is that gay people aren't always so eager to identify themselves. Another is deciding who counts. Do you count only people who identify as gay and are—or have been—sexually active? Do you count people who simply identify as gay? Or do you count everyone who has ever had a homosexual experience?

One of the more interesting studies I read was published in 1993 by the University of Chicago Press under the title *The Social Organization of Sexuality.* The study found that the percentage of gay men and women in the U.S. population varied widely between the big cities, the suburbs, and rural areas. For example, in the top twelve largest cities, 10.2 percent of the men and 2.1 percent of the women reported having had a sexual partner of their own gender in the previous year. In the suburbs of the top twelve cities, 2.7 percent of the men and 1.2 percent of the women reported having had a sexual partner of their own gender in the previous year. And for rural areas, the figures were 1.0 percent for men and 0.6 percent for women.

My educated guess is that approximately 3 percent of men and about half that number of women have same-gender sexual orientation, whether or not they express it by having a relationship of some kind with a person of the same gender. But whatever the actual figures, there are undoubtedly tens of millions of gay and lesbian people around the world.

As far as the reasons for the difference between the number of gay men and the number of lesbians goes—it is a mystery that remains to be solved.

Have there always been gay people?

Homosexuality and homosexual behavior are not modern inventions, as is evident from historical writings and from depictions of homosexual behavior in ancient art.

Are there are a lot more gay people now than in the past?

This is a question my grandmother asked me. She told me that she remembered back in the 1940s seeing a man on the subway platform in her Brooklyn, New York, neighborhood who "held his cigarette a certain way, wore makeup, and dressed impeccably."

Because of this man's manner and clothing, she just assumed he was gay, based on the stereotype with which she was familiar. "Now you see gay people on television, read about them in the newspaper, and they have parades. Where did they all come from?" she asked.

Gay and lesbian people have always been a part of the population, but because most gay men and women look and act just like most nongay people, there was no way for my grandmother to know that there were other gay men and lesbians on the subway platform with her in addition to the one man she assumed was gay. The difference today is that many gay people no longer feel compelled to hide their sexual orientation, and they live their lives like everyone else. So it just seems like there are more gay people.

? Do animals other than humans engage in homosexual behavior?

Scientists have observed consistent homosexual behavior in the animal kingdom in many different species, ranging from mountain rams and seagulls to gorillas. No one has yet suggested that this is the result of a passive father and a domineering mother.

? Is homosexuality nature's way of controlling the population?

If that is Mother Nature's purpose, she hasn't succeeded, primarily because many, if not most, gay and lesbian people—even to this day—hide their feelings of sexual attraction, enter heterosexual marriages, and have children. Besides which, a growing number of openly gay and lesbian individuals and couples are choosing to have children.

? What are some common stereotypes about gay men and lesbians? Do gay men have better fashion and design sense than straight men? Are lesbians better athletes than straight women? Do all lesbians have cats? Do gay men lisp? Why don't lesbians wear makeup?

Stereotypes don't come completely out of nowhere, so I would be willing to bet that a greater percentage of gay men have better fashion and design sense than straight men. But this is certainly not a universal trait.

Over the years, because of my work, I've interviewed gay people in their homes across the country. And most often, their fashion and design sense is nothing to write home about—and that's the case with lesbians and gay men just about equally. I might add that when I needed to buy clothes recently, I was helped in my choices by two lesbians who have far better fashion and design sense than I do.

As far as the other stereotypes I've listed in the above questions, well, no one has done a study as to whether lesbians make better athletes than straight women, have more cats than the average straight woman, or wear more or less makeup. But my guess is that if the marketing geniuses who have figured out how to sell expensive shampoo to children think that lesbians own more cats than other women, then they'll find a way to identify and quantify that market and then create products and advertising that will get lesbians to buy more, and more expensive, cat food.

And if gay men do indeed have speech impediments more frequently than straight men, speech therapists ought to think about advertising their services in publications and on Web sites that reach gay men. (I think they'd be wasting their money.)

? Do gay men hate women? Do lesbians hate men?

Everyone is capable of hating, no matter what his or her sexual orientation or gender. But as a rule, no, gay men don't hate women, and lesbians don't hate men.

? Do gay men and women hate straight people?

Some gay and lesbian people have hostile feelings toward heterosexual people. This should come as no surprise, given some of the terrible things gay people have experienced at the hands of some straight people. But as a rule, no, gay people don't hate straight people.

? What does "GLBT," "LGBT," and "GLBTQ" stand for?

These are acronyms that you'll see used frequently in print to describe the increasingly diverse group of people who come under the umbrella of gay rights efforts and gay organizations. Here's what they stand for:

GLBT = gay, lesbian, bisexual, and transgender

LGBT = lesbian, gay, bisexual, and transgender

GLBTQ = gay, lesbian, bisexual, transgender, and queer; *or* gay, lesbian, bisexual, transgender, and questioning youth

What do gay people like to be called?

Most gay people would like to be called by their given names. Regarding their sexual orientation, if you asked the average gay man, he would tell you that he prefers the word "gay." If you asked the average gay woman, she would tell you that she prefers "gay" or "lesbian."

Some gay people prefer to call themselves "queer" and find it liberating to embrace a word that was once used as a slur against homosexuals. They also find the word inclusive in comparison to gay, lesbian, bisexual, and so forth.

What does the word "faggot" mean? What does the word "dyke" mean?

These are words that most gay people do not like being called. Let's start with "faggot," or its abbreviated relative, "fag." These words have evolved into general-purpose put-downs, wielded usually by young people against those they perceive to be stupid, dorky, weird, weak, etc. While "fag" and "faggot" are most often used against boys, they're now used against girls, too.

Back in the 1970s, when I was a kid, "faggot" was a term of contempt used against those boys and men who were perceived to be homosexuals and/or less than masculine. And long before that, the word "faggot" was used to describe a bundle of sticks, twigs, or branches used for fuel. (I remember that when I was in college some of the more worldly smokers referred to cigarettes as fags, as in, "I desperately need a fag.")

The word "dyke" is not nearly as versatile and is gender-specific. It's most often used as a disparaging term for lesbians, particularly those who are perceived to be masculine. It is also used against women—gay or straight—who refuse to conform to society's expectations in terms of how they look and act.

For more information on these two words, visit the GLSEN Web site, which offers a school lesson plan devoted to this subject: www.glsen.com.

Why do some gay people call themselves "fags" and "dykes"?

Like other minority groups, some gay and lesbian people playfully use words that are used by the larger population to put them down. Some say it's a way of taking the sting out of those words. (I think it's stupid, insulting, and degrading. But that's just my opinion.)

Bear in mind that you can use these words playfully only if you yourself are gay or lesbian. There are, however, exceptions. One of my gay male friends is not at all bothered when his heterosexual women friends use the word "fag" while in his company. He knows they're simply being playful and is not at all bothered by it.

Is there a gay and lesbian culture?

I thought I'd offer an explanation of gay culture given to me by the late Chuck Rowland, one of eight founders of the Mattachine Society, a gay rights organization started in Los Angeles in 1950 (which marked the birth of the gay rights movement in the United States). Rowland was one of the first people to argue that there was a distinct gay and lesbian culture.

When I interviewed Rowland in 1989, he told me that he had an especially hard time in the 1950s explaining to other gay people what he meant by *gay culture.* He said, "People would say, 'Do you actually think we're more cultured than anybody else?' I would explain that I was using *culture* in the sociological sense—as a body of language, feelings, thinking, experiences that we share in common. As we speak of a Mexican culture. As we speak of an American Indian culture."

In the decades since Chuck Rowland first made his case for the existence of gay culture, gay and lesbian writers, artists, photographers, playwrights, choreographers, filmmakers, and so forth have created a very significant body of work for gay and lesbian people that we would normally associate with the cultural life of a community.

2

Growing Up

? At what age do you know you're gay?

First, a story. My friend Stephanie was ferrying her six-year-old son and two of his friends between school and tumbling class when she heard one of the boys raise the subject of marriage and question whether one of the other boys was going to marry a boy or a girl. Stephanie recalled, "After some back-and-forth he said he was going to marry a girl. Then the boy sitting in the middle said, 'I'm definitely marrying a boy.' I just about drove off the road. Not because I think there's anything wrong with gay people—my brother is gay and happily coupled—but this boy was so emphatic. He just knew. And then my son chimed in with his declaration that he was going to marry a girl. And that was that. They were so matter-of-fact about it and then went right on to the next subject."

Thc six-year-old who knew he was going to marry a boy is years away from puberty and from having strong feelings of sexual attraction, but he's already imagining a future that is different from what his friends are imagining. It's probably a little early to say that he's going to grow up to be a gay kid, but it wouldn't be at all surprising. A lot of gay and lesbian adults I've talk to and interviewed over the years recalled having "known" at five or six years of age that they were gay, whether or not they fully understood or had a word for what they were feeling.

That was Deborah's experience. She knew from early childhood that she was different from other girls: "I was supposed to be sweet and docile, but I was a jock. I wanted to grab the world by the balls! And I had sexual feelings very, very early, but boys were not an interest.

"When the other little girls were starting to get crushes on boys and were talking about weddings, I always knew I wanted to marry a girl—always, always, always. When I was seven, I remember telling my parents that I was not going to marry a man and all the reasons why. By the time I was ten, I explained to them that I was in love with this little girl. My dad told me that it was just a phase; that I was going to outgrow it."

Young kids and even teenagers have crushes on friends of the same gender, and it doesn't necessarily mean that they're gay. But for Deborah, the crushes were no passing thing. What proved confusing for her was that until she was cast in the play *The Children's Hour* in the seventh grade, she didn't know about lesbians. "That's when I learned about women with women," she told me. "I was doing a scene with this woman I had a serious crush on, and she got to the part where she explained how she really felt for her female coworker. It hit me like a ton of bricks: 'That's what this is!' "

People who have feelings of sexual attraction for the same gender become aware of these feelings at the same time that all people become aware of their feelings of attraction, whether that's from earliest conscious memory, as it was for Deborah, or during preadolescence or adolescence, or later. But there are differences.

For heterosexual people, these feelings of attraction are reinforced by family, society, culture, and religion from the earliest age. For example, how many times have you heard loving relatives ask a young child if he has a girlfriend or she has a boyfriend? Even if it's asked in the most playful way, this question reinforces the idea that boys have girlfriends and girls have boyfriends.

For a gay or lesbian child growing up, the experience is very different. Even before they're fully aware of their feelings of attraction or the implications of those feelings, gay and lesbian kids generally know that what they're feeling isn't how things are supposed to be. And depending upon what they hear from their parents and those around them, they may learn very quickly not to share their fantasies about the gender of the person they plan to marry when they grow up.

? Can you discover that you're gay later in life?

Every human being's experience of his or her sexual orientation and sexuality is different. Though most people have a strong sense of their feelings of sexual attraction by the time they're adolescents, there are people—primarily women—for whom the full range or full complexity of these feelings don't become clear or emerge until they reach their thirties or forties.

I've included this specific question because I heard from a woman via e-mail who read an earlier edition of this book and thought that this was a subject I failed to adequately address.

Here's an excerpt of what she wrote to me:

> *There are people like me who did not "become gay" until later in life. Since I myself have no idea why it happened I can't explain this to my mother. I just know that since I have*

started having relationships with other women I am more comfortable and happier than I ever was with a man in every way imaginable.

If I understand your book correctly, you are saying that the fact that I was not sexually attracted to women for twenty-six years means I was straight. (I don't argue that.) I am not now, nor have I in the last five years had any desire for a relationship with a man, which would mean I am gay. (I don't argue that, either.)

However, you left no room in your book for this transition and decidedly dramatic change to take place later in life and I am afraid it will only confirm my mother's belief that you are either born gay or you are not and that I must be straight because I was not born gay.

The letter was signed "Late Bloomer."

I hope I haven't given the impression that I think we are born gay or straight. What I believe is that we are given our innate feelings of sexual attraction extremely early in life—before birth or after—and these feelings are our own.

For some people these feelings are entirely straightforward, as they were for my brother and me. We both had a clear sense early on of what our feelings were and what we preferred. That's not everyone's experience. And for some people, feelings of sexual attraction may leave room for a range of experiences and the discovery of feelings later in life that they may not have recognized were there. This was the case for "Late Bloomer."

? Do gay people feel bad or embarrassed about being gay?

I did. It was not uncommon for gay people to feel that way during the years in which I grew up, when there were virtually no positive gay images or role models. I thought my life was over. How could I be something that was considered so disgusting, so loathsome, so awful? How could I be what people called a homo, a queer, a sissy, a fag? What I didn't know until later was that feeling bad about my attraction to men (a very few men, I might add) was a perfectly normal reaction to what I had learned from the world around me about homosexuals and the life I could expect to lead.

When I got to college and started meeting other gay and lesbian people, I was surprised to discover that there were kids who didn't feel at all bad or embarrassed about being gay. They knew from when they were very young that what they felt was normal for them, and they didn't care what anybody else thought. I admired them then, and still admire them now for their fortitude in the face of what was then an almost uniformly hostile society.

In more recent years, as gay and lesbian people have become increasingly visible and parents have learned to be supportive and accepting of their gay kids early on, the experience of growing up gay for many boys and girls and young men and women has been getting easier. I like to think that the majority of this generation's gay kids and young adults will be spared the experience of feeling bad about themselves or hating themselves because they're gay.

I still get plenty of e-mails from gay kids and teens who are struggling with bad feelings about their sexual orientation—especially from young people who live in countries where homosexuality remains a taboo subject or a crime—but I also hear from a lot of kids who feel good about themselves, know they can count on their parents and friends to accept, love, and support them, and anticipate lives that are no different from anyone else's.

? How do gay people learn to accept that they are gay or lesbian?

For some people it's automatic, but for most it's a process, and people learn to accept themselves through a variety of means. They may do their own personal research, reading everything they can find on the subject of homosexuality, or they may find role models in their families or communities.

They may join support groups for gay and lesbian youth, or they may attend meetings organized by their high school's gay-straight alliance, or GSA. (Hundreds of high schools and a handful of middle schools across the county have such groups. See chapter 15, "Education," for more on GSAs.) And some people see a school counselor or a private therapist who can help them learn to accept their sexual orientation.

Not everyone who is gay or lesbian accepts their feelings of sexual attraction and may in fact work very hard at trying to repress or get rid of these feelings. Some people search for a "cure" through therapy, religion, or an organization that promises to show them "the way out of the homosexual lifestyle." There is, of course, no cure for homosexuality, because it's not a disease any more than is heterosexuality. And anyone or any organization that offers a cure or tells you that you can change your innate feelings of sexual attraction is lying.

? Do gay men and lesbians like being gay?

I put this question to several gay and lesbian people, and they offered several different responses. Among those who like being gay, some people said they can't imagine being any different. Others feel that they're more sensitive and more insightful people because of their experience of growing up in a world where they're outsiders. Others feel lucky to have been given the opportunity to question life's assumptions and to consider what they really wanted from life without automatically progressing from single life to marriage to children.

Those people I spoke with who had negative feelings about being gay also offered a variety of reasons for their feelings. Some said they would have had better luck finding a spouse if they had been heterosexual, or that being gay has held them back in their careers, or that being gay has made it difficult to have children.

What's it like to be a gay kid or teenager?

Everyone's experience is different, but in general, growing up gay or lesbian is challenging for most gay kids and teenagers. In some ways things are quite different from when I was a teenager, because now there are many resources for gay kids, particularly online, and the subject of homosexuality is so openly discussed and debated. But in other ways, from what I hear, things aren't very different, especially the ease with which kids use put-downs like "fag" and "Don't be so gay."

I have only a handful of vivid memories from when I was just beginning to come to terms with being gay. One of those memories is from a Sunday-afternoon party in the spring of 1976, during my senior year at Hillcrest High School in New York City. About twenty of us were scattered around the living room of a friend's apartment.

Across from where I was standing, my friend Ruth was sitting on a big easy chair, with her boyfriend on one arm of the chair and our mutual friend Dave on the other. I was pretty sure by then that Dave was gay; we'd started dropping hints to each other a few weeks before. (We'd even admitted to each other that we might be bisexual.)

Everyone was listening to Ruth, who somehow worked her way onto the subject of gay people and declared, "I guess it's okay with me, but I wouldn't want one of them near me." Instantly, Dave and I locked eyes. Ruth had no idea that the man sitting next to her was gay (after we graduated, Dave told me he was gay) and that the friend who picked her up every day for three years to go to school—me!—was also gay. "What would she think?" I wondered. "Would she still want to be my friend?"

The two emotions that most dominated my life at that time were fear and a sense of isolation. I was fearful of what my friends and family would think of me if they knew the truth, and I felt enormous isolation, because there was no one I could talk to. This is one of the reasons that when I hear from gay people who have told no one but me the truth about their sexual orientation, I urge them to find people they can talk to. I know from personal experience how awful and damaging such isolation can be.

Contrary to my own experience is that of a young woman who wrote to me a few years ago. Tammy, who is now in her twenties, found a group of supportive friends—gay and nongay—on her high school volleyball team. "I always knew I was lucky to have a group of friends I didn't have to keep secrets from when I was that young," she said, "It really helped me accept being gay.

"There were a couple of other lesbians on the team, and we were all out to each other and the rest of the team. I don't know, maybe it was just the right time or it was the right group of people, or maybe it's finally sinking in that there's nothing wrong with us."

? If you can't talk to your parents or friends and you think you're gay, whom can you talk to? Where can you get information? Are there organizations for gay young people?

If you think you're gay, lesbian, bisexual, or whatever, find someone you can trust—and talk to them. You'll feel better if you share what you're thinking with someone else. If there isn't anyone in your life you can trust—a best friend, a sibling, a school counselor—you have other options. In many cities there are gay, lesbian, bisexual, and transgender youth groups, and across the country there are hundreds of local organizations that provide a range of services to gay youth. In addition, hundreds of high schools and some middle schools have gay-straight alliances (GSAs).

The best place to start your research is the National Youth Advocacy Coalition (NYAC). In addition to providing extensive information for gay, lesbian, bisexual, transgender, and questioning young people, the NYAC Web site (www.nyacyouth.org) lists state-by-state resources. And the Gay, Lesbian and Straight Education Network (GLSEN) offers state-by-state information about GSAs on its Web site (www.glsen.org).

Another organization I recommend for gay young people is Parents, Families and Friends of Lesbians and Gays (PFLAG). At a local PFLAG chapter or through the organization's Web site (www.pflag.org) you can find an accepting mom or dad who has lots of experience with this issue and will be more than happy to talk to you.

? What do straight kids and teens think of their gay and lesbian peers?

Straight kids have a whole range of responses to their gay and lesbian peers, from easy acceptance to thoughts and acts of physical violence. And no one knows better than gay teens themselves what other kids think of them, because the vast majority of gay students report being "verbally, sexually, or physically harassed because of their sexual orientation"—this according to GLSEN's "National School Climate Survey." (For the full report, visit GLSEN's Web site: www.glsen.org.)

But what straight kids and teens feel toward their gay peers can be exceedingly complex. For example, one woman I spoke with who has traveled to New York City high school classrooms to educate students about gay and lesbian people offered an interesting perspective. She told me, "Many of these heterosexual teenagers are furious at their gay and lesbian peers for hiding. They think they're liars and cheats and deceivers and manipulators.

"But the fact is, these gay and lesbian kids are afraid—mostly of being rejected. So when you explain to teenagers what's really going on—that these gay and lesbian kids are not being criminals or betrayers—and explain how much pain and terror they're experiencing, then they say, 'Oh, I get it. I didn't want to be mean to that person for that.'

"I also tell these kids, 'It's up to you to make the first move. Do not expect your gay and lesbian friends to come to you and tell you they're gay if you have not given them a signal that it's okay to talk to you."

? What do kids learn in school about homosexuality?

See chapter 15, "Education."

? Do gay teens take their boyfriends and girlfriends to high school proms? Why? Why not?

Most gay and lesbian teens who choose to attend their high school prom either go with a group of friends or take an opposite-gender date, and they do so for several reasons: They may not yet have come to terms with their sexual orientation or aren't fully aware of these feelings, so they wouldn't think of taking a same-gender date to the prom. They don't want the other students to know they're gay. They're fearful of how other students will react. They don't want their parents to find out that they're gay or lesbian. They don't want to be the focus of attention, which a same-gender couple most certainly will be. Or they don't want to get in trouble with their school's administration.

The earliest stories I came across about high school students taking same-gender dates to proms involved two young men at a high school in Medford, Massachusetts, in 1975, and two young women at Girls High in Philadelphia in 1976. Through the years, some students who have brought same-gender dates to proms have been welcomed, and others have had to fight school administrators in court.

Those gay kids who choose to take a same-gender date to a high school prom generally do so for the same reasons that heterosexual teenagers do: because they want to go with a date of their choice. As Aaron Fricke wrote in 1980 in his landmark book *Reflections of a Rock Lobster,* about his experience of having to sue his high school in Cumberland, Rhode Island, in order to bring his male date: "The simple, obvious thing would have been to go to the senior prom with a girl. But that would have been a lie—a lie to myself, to the girl, and to all the other students. What I *wanted* to do was to take a male date."

Beyond a desire to be true to himself, Fricke also wanted to make a larger point. He wrote: "I concluded that taking a guy to the prom would be a strong positive statement about the existence of gay people. Any opposition to my case (and I anticipated a good bit) would show the negative side of society—not homosexuality."

3

Coming Out / Going Public

? What does "coming out" or "coming out of the closet" mean?

To explain how a gay or lesbian person "comes out of the closet," you first need to know what "the closet" is. The closet is simply a metaphor used to describe the place where many gay and lesbian people keep their sexual orientation hidden—whether that place is between their ears, within a tightly knit group of friends, or within the larger gay and lesbian community. The truth is kept "in the closet," with the door closed.

At its most basic, "coming out of the closet" means being honest with those around you—friends, family, colleagues, and so forth—about your sexual orientation, about who you are. For example, it could be something as simple as speaking in a matter-of-fact way about your same-gender partner if a new colleague asks you if you're married.

Coming out of the closet means different things to different people. When you ask three different gay and lesbian people to talk about their coming-out experiences, you're likely to get three entirely different stories. One person may talk about coming out sexually—his or her first sexual experience. Another may talk about coming out to herself—when she first accepted the fact that she was a lesbian. Still another will talk about coming out to his family—when he first told his family he was gay.

? Heterosexuals don't "come out," so why do gay people?

Straight people don't have to come out of the closet, because they've never been in one. They've never been compelled to lie about or hide their sexual orientation, because they live in a society that accepts and celebrates it.

Growing up, heterosexual boys and girls think nothing of talking about a crush on a friend, rock star, or favorite actor or actress. When they're old enough to date, they can introduce their opposite-gender romantic interest to their friends and parents, and they can hold hands with that person while walking down the street. At work, they can speak freely about their girlfriend, boyfriend, husband, or wife without fear of losing their job. They can put a picture of a spouse on their desk with no questions asked. They have no need to let people know in a specific way what their sexual orientation is, because their actions and words over time let everyone know that they're heterosexual.

Most gay and lesbian people grow up hiding their thoughts, crushes, and relationships. Typically, they enter adolescence or young adulthood with the closely held secret that they're gay or lesbian. Some have gone to great lengths to hide their secret, perhaps dating opposite-gender partners or even marrying. Eventually, many gay men and women choose to reveal the truth about their sexual orientation, but because they've kept that part of their lives secret up until that point, disclosure occurs all at once and may come as a shock to friends and loved ones.

I look forward to the day when all kids growing up feel no need to hide their true feelings, a day when gay and lesbian kids have no need to come out of the closet because they've never been in one.

Why can't gay people just keep it to themselves?

Easier said than done. Have you ever had a secret? Even a small one? Then try to imagine what it would be like to keep a really, really big secret like your sexual orientation.

Imagine that it's Monday morning at the office, and one of your colleagues asks you what you did for the weekend. You answer, as you always do, "Nothing much," even though you spent the weekend at the hospital with your seriously ill spouse. You could have said that you spent the weekend in the hospital with a person close to you, but more questions would inevitably follow, and ultimately it would be impossible to hide the truth. So to protect your secret, you almost never honestly respond to an innocent question or comment, whether the question is asked by a colleague, relative, or even a cab driver. You have to monitor everything you say.

As a test, just take note during an average day of how many times your personal life comes up in conversation, whether you're at a mall buying clothes or on an airplane seated next to a chatty stranger. Imagine how you would respond if you had to hide this key fact of your life.

Those gay and lesbian people who choose to tell their friends, family, and colleagues about their sexual orientation do so for many reasons. However, they do it primarily because they want to be themselves, because they want to be honest with those they love and trust, and because it can be difficult, exhausting, and personally destructive to pretend to be someone you're not.

Why do some gay people choose to stay in the closet and hide their sexual orientation?

Gay and lesbian people stay in the closet for three primary reasons: necessity, fear, and because they simply prefer or are accustomed to discussing this part of their lives with only a select group of people.

Those who stay in the closet because of necessity or fear may do so because they know, suspect, or fear they'll lose their jobs or compromise their careers, that their parents will stop paying their college tuition or throw them out of the house if they find out, that they'll lose custody of their children, be harshly judged by the people around them, or subjected to physical violence at the hands of those who hate gay people.

What's it like for gay people who hide their sexual orientation?

"It's exhausting and frightening," said Beverly, who spent more than a dozen years in the military hiding the fact that she was a lesbian. "I never knew when the ax would fall, when someone would turn me in. At any moment I knew my career could be over. So I watched everything I said, everything I did, to make sure no one would guess the truth. I tell you, it was the hardest thing I ever did in my life. I thought I was going to lose my mind."

Keeping your sexual orientation hidden means living—and remembering—two different lives: your real life, and a semifictional life that's suitable for public consumption. You have to monitor what you say and be careful of what you do, and you have to make certain your two lives never intersect.

When you attend public functions, you'll likely need to bring a date of the opposite gender, even if you've been living with your same-gender partner for twenty years. When your kids visit you and your same-gender spouse for the weekend, you have to pretend that you're roommates and make certain you've left no incriminating evidence—a book or magazine, for example—anywhere in the house. (Kids are curious, and if there's something to be found, they'll find it.) Above all, you've got to be an expert storyteller, and you've got to be able to tell a convincing lie with a straight face.

When I was a teenager, I was terrified that people would find out I was gay, because I couldn't imagine I'd ever be accepted or as highly regarded if the people most important to me knew the truth. So I worked hard to keep my secret, and I made up all kinds of stories to cover my tracks.

Once when I was home on vacation during my first year in college, I went out with some gay friends on a Friday night. I told my mother a story about where I was going and with whom. And I told my girlfriend from high school, who was also home from college, something about having gone to a party.

I didn't mean to tell two different stories, but I couldn't remember what I'd told my mother. So there we all were the next evening, the three of us, in the living room at my mother's house, and Eileen asks me how my Friday night party had been. Well, I couldn't remember what story I'd told my mother, but it was clear from the expression on her face that I hadn't told her I was at a party. Eileen saw the expression on my mother's face and the look of horror on my face, and there was a split second when everyone realized I'd been caught in a lie.

It was in that awful moment in my mother's living room that I realized I didn't have the talent, the memory, or the true desire required to keep my life a secret. I was a failure at staying in the closet. Fortunately, I have a family that accepts me as I am and a career that doesn't require me to hide. Actually, I chose a career that requires me to be quite open.

Many people are experts at keeping their homosexuality carefully hidden and don't find it especially difficult. For example, Tom is in his late fifties, in a relationship with a man for more than a quarter century, and deep in the closet to everyone but his close circle of gay male friends. As far as his colleagues know, he's a confirmed bachelor who has no life beyond his career.

Tom explains: "I learned a long time ago how to keep my two worlds—my personal life and my professional life—entirely separate. I never socialize with people from work and never discuss anything about my personal life with my colleagues. My partner and I have separate phones at home, both of which are unlisted, so even if someone suspected I had a male spouse, they could never trace us through the phone company.

"Given the times through which I've lived, I would never have gotten as far as I have in my career if it were known that I'm gay, and I'm not about to risk all I have just so I can bring my partner to company parties. It's not worth it.

"Years ago, when I was growing up, there was no choice. No one ever talked about coming out of the closet, because it would have been such an outrageous thing to do. Only crazy people didn't hide. You *had* to keep it hidden. Now there's a choice, but I'm happy and very comfortable with the way I live my life."

The challenge for people like Tom, as it is for all gay people who wish to keep their sexual orientation hidden, is that as openly gay people have become more commonplace and the issue of gay rights remains part of the national political agenda, it's increasingly difficult to fool people about your sexual orientation.

? When do gay people come out of the closet?

I know a woman who at the age of seven told her parents that she wanted to marry another girl. I don't know if you would call this coming out of the closet, but she certainly alarmed her parents. And I know a man who didn't tell another soul he was gay until he was nearly eighty-five.

More typically, those gay and lesbian people who choose to live their lives openly start sharing the truth about their sexual orientation with friends, family, classmates, and colleagues from their teens through their twenties.

? How do you do it?

There are many different ways to let people know you're gay. Some people write letters or e-mails to their parents or friends, discuss it by phone, or do it face-to-face in conversation. (Just a cautionary note here if you're planning to disclose your sexual orientation in an e-mail or instant message. Anything sent electronically can find its way from your mailbox to hundreds of other mailboxes in the blink of an eye. So if you would like to maintain some control over who knows and who doesn't, I highly recommend restricting yourself to paper letters, phone conversations—on a land line if you want to be really careful—and face-to-face discussions.)

Other people who want to come out drop hints, hoping that someone will ask a question that will give them an opportunity to answer truthfully. Still others, celebrities in particular, come out in their published autobiographies, go on television talk shows, or talk about their sexual orientation in magazine interviews. Whatever the choice, the decision to come out is likely one that a gay or lesbian person has thought about and possibly agonized over for a long time.

The Human Rights Campaign, as part of its National Coming Out Project, provides coming out information on its Web site (www.hrc.org/comingout) geared for lesbian, gay, bisexual, and transgender young people and their parents. The information includes resources for coming out in the African-American, Hispanic, and Asian Pacific communities.

? Do you come out just once?

Unless you're a well-recognized celebrity or high-level politician, coming out is not something you do just once and then forget about. For gay and lesbian people who choose to live their lives openly, coming out is something you may wind up doing almost every day. Here's why: there are all kinds of chance encounters and conversations that force gay people to decide whether to answer honestly.

For example, every now and then my partner and I are asked if we're brothers. I don't think we look like brothers, not even close, but people generally recognize that there is a closeness to our relationship and the way we interact that suggests we're something more than just friends. When that happens, we have to decide whether to simply answer no, or to go into more detail.

At the grocery store, the first time we were asked by a checkout clerk if we were brothers, I simply said no. Then I was mad at myself for days afterward for not having done what any heterosexual couple would have done if they'd been asked if they were brother and sister, which would have been to say, "No, we're a couple" or "No, we're married." So the next time we encountered a curious checkout clerk, I said we were a couple and that was that.

Recently, while on vacation, we were talking with the twelve-year-old son of a couple who were vacationing at the same small hotel where we were spending the Christmas holiday. From an earlier conversation, he knew we both worked in the publishing business, and his favorite books were the topic of this conversation.

During a pause in our discussion, he asked, "So, are you brothers?" It was clear that the boy was trying to figure out our relationship. I answered simply, and in what I thought was an age-appropriate way, by telling him we were partners. "Oh, do you work together?" he asked. "No," I said, "we live together." "Are you roommates?" he asked. And with that question I realized I needed to be clear, especially because it seemed apparent that he was looking for specific confirmation of what he already suspected. So I said, "We're a couple, just like your mom and dad." His response? "Oh, that's cool."

Not all gay people have to say anything to let people know that they're gay. Dave and Judy, best friends and neighbors for more than ten years, told me they never have to tell anyone that they're gay. "We couldn't pass for straight in this lifetime," said

Judy, "no matter how hard we tried. We're living proof that the gay stereotype came from somewhere."

Dave is slight, has delicate features, and is very effeminate. Judy is a self-described "big butch." She's built like a construction worker, is partial to jeans and sweatshirts, and has a deep voice. "We're always getting hassled," said Dave, "because people can tell. Sometimes we envy people who can pass, but in a lot of ways it's easier for us. Because we can't hide, we've never had to worry about coming out. We were out before we even knew what we were."

? What does it feel like to come out?

I can't speak for all gay and lesbian people, but virtually all of the hundreds of gay men and lesbians I've interviewed over the years have told me that coming out has ultimately been a positive and liberating experience. And that includes people who have lost their jobs and those who've been rejected by their families, even by their children. The experience of coming out may have been painful, frightening, overwhelming, or even traumatic, but none of the people I've spoken with have said they regret leaving the secrets behind and living their lives openly.

Here's just one example, although it's not typical, since most people don't come out on national television. Gary, who grew up in a very small southwestern town, came out of the closet to his family, friends, and colleagues when he was a guest on a network television talk show on National Coming Out Day. (Regarding National Coming Out Day, see the last question in this chapter.)

As scared as Gary was of how the people in his life would react, especially his parents, he said he felt an incredible sense of relief and renewal. "It was like being born," he said. "It was the first time I stood up and said, 'This is who I am, and I'm proud of who I am.' The burden had been lifted from my shoulders. For the first time I felt like I had a life.

"For someone who was always embarrassed about being gay, that wasn't easy, especially on national television. And it took me until I was thirty-five to do it. But it was important for me to do it for myself and to set an example for young people, to show them that there's a better way, that you don't have to hide the way I did and waste all those years.

"My only regret about the whole experience was that I hadn't done it sooner. Of course, I felt bad about upsetting my parents, but it had been on my shoulders since I was a kid. It was time for them to deal with it. It wasn't my problem anymore."

? Why is it such a big deal for gay people to come out to their parents?

It's such a big deal because there's potentially so much at stake. It's not exactly like telling your parents you got an "F" in math. People generally know their parents well enough to know how they'll react to a bad grade. But no matter how well people think they know their parents, few feel absolutely certain of how their parents will respond to the news that their child is gay. And it's that fear—the fear of the unknown—that keeps people from speaking with their parents and causes most gay people so much anxiety even when they anticipate such a conversation.

And it's not for no reason that gay people worry about how their parents will respond. Everyone has heard stories of parents who have withdrawn their love or financial support, thrown their kids out of the house, or just cried a lot. And who wants to make their parents cry?

I have one friend who moved halfway around the world when he was in his early twenties, in large part just to avoid the possibility of his parents finding out he was gay. He'd convinced himself he was protecting his parents from news that he knew would at best disappoint them, and at worst—well, he didn't dare imagine how bad it could be, even if a really bad reaction was inconsistent with who he knew his parents to be.

After eight years abroad, my friend returned home for good, knowing that he had to tell his parents the truth about his life. "I'm really close to my parents," he said, "so this wasn't something I could continue to hide from them. But it wasn't until I'd gotten a good job and was sure I could stand on my own two feet that I finally told them. My dad was instantly fine with it. My mum took a little longer. But basically they've been great, and our relationship is better than it's been since . . . well, better than it's ever been."

Another example: Michelle, an accountant in her late twenties who lives in Atlanta, finally told her parents she was a lesbian, after thinking about doing it for nearly ten years. "At first I couldn't get past the fear they would reject me," she said. "When I was still living at home, I thought they'd throw me out of the house. Then I was afraid they'd pull me out of college. After college I was still afraid they would reject me, but that was compounded by my fear that I'd disappoint them; they had always been so proud of my accomplishments.

"I never liked keeping secrets from my parents, but I didn't find it terribly difficult as long as I wasn't dating anyone. But then I fell in love and began a serious relationship. There was so much I wanted to tell my parents, but all we wound up talking about was the weather and the cows. (My parents are dairy farmers.) I knew they were worried about me being alone, but if I told them I wasn't alone and that my roommate was more than just my roommate, I was afraid of destroying their lives.

"Finally I got up my courage to tell them. It was so hard to say the words, but it was an incredible relief to finally have it out in the open. That was several years ago now, and my parents are doing okay. It's not easy for them to talk about it, but they're making a good effort."

? Are there some people who don't tell their parents that they're gay?

Of course, especially people who have parents who they know cannot accept them. This is more typically the case with deeply religious parents, but there are also parents who are not deeply religious but come from traditional cultures in which homosexuality is also unacceptable.

I'm reluctant to make a blanket statement here that all such parents can never accept their gay children, because this is not the case. But gay people who have parents they suspect will reject them or worse must be extremely careful in considering whether it's in their best interest to reveal their sexual orientation.

And it's not just people who have parents they know will reject them who choose not to discuss their homosexuality. For example, Steve, who is in his late thirties, doesn't think his parents will reject him. He simply doesn't have much of a relationship with them. He said, "I've never discussed anything personal with my parents about any aspect of my life, so why would I talk about this? Besides, they live halfway across the country, so I only see them once or twice a year. Why make trouble and why burden them when it won't accomplish anything?"

Steve resents the pressure some of his friends have put on him to tell his parents the truth. "It's my choice," he said, "and it works for me. There's no law that says I have to come out to them if I don't want to. If I thought it would make my life better, I'd think about it. Some of my friends say I would have a closer relationship with my parents if I told them, but I don't want a closer relationship with them."

? If you're gay and you would like to come out to your parents, what should you do?

You've got a lot of homework to do before you talk to your parents about being gay, because in all likelihood you're going to have to be the expert for your parents on this subject. Most parents, unless they're gay themselves, will likely have a lot of questions, and this is not a situation where you want to get caught struggling for answers. So the first thing you should do is make use of the resources offered by two key national gay rights groups.

First, the Human Rights Campaign's National Coming Out Project offers lots of information on this subject (www.hrc.org/comingout). And this includes information specific to the African-American, Hispanic, and Asian Pacific communities.

Second, visit the Web site for Parents, Families and Friends of Lesbians and Gays (www.pflag.org). PFLAG is a national nonprofit organization with hundreds of affiliate groups across the United States. You'll find lots of information on PFLAG's Web site about what you need to consider before talking to your parents, what you can expect from them if you do, the questions they're likely to have, and the answers you'll need. Through the Web site you can also locate and contact the nearest PFLAG affiliate group and talk to knowledgeable parents who can advise you on how to handle your specific circumstances. (See the "Resources" section at the back of this book for complete contact information.)

You might also consider talking to a school counselor or therapist who has experience dealing in an affirmative way with gay people. A counselor can help you sort out your thoughts, explore all the issues you need to consider in advance of speaking with your parents, and then provide support in the aftermath.

? If your child comes out to you, what should you say?

See chapter 5, "For Parents of Gay Children."

? Why do some people who have been married for years to someone of the opposite sex suddenly come out of the closet and say they're gay? Have they always been gay?

This question came to me from a woman whose husband came out to her after twenty-five years of marriage. She could not understand why her husband didn't tell her sooner or keep the secret until he died.

From having interviewed men and women who come out after many years of heterosexual marriage, I know that the decision to come out to a heterosexual spouse is most often an extremely difficult one. And the decision to do so is made because the gay spouse can no longer keep their secret.

There are many reasons why a gay spouse can no longer continue in a heterosexual marriage. For example, they may be unable to continue living with the burden of such a large secret, they may wish to find a same-gender partner, or they may have already fallen in love with someone of the same gender.

Whether the "newly gay" spouse has always been aware of his or her feelings depends upon the individual. What *is* clear is that they've always had feelings of sexual attraction for people of the same gender. However, while some men and women are fully aware of these feelings, others have suppressed them, and still others have come to understand these feelings only later in life.

This is an extremely complicated and emotional issue, particularly for the straight spouses left behind, and it deserves far more discussion than the brief answer I can provide here. So first I suggest that you take a look at the related questions in chapter 6, "Dating, Relationships, and Marriage." And then visit the Web site for the Straight Spouse Network (www.ssnetwk.org). I also highly recommend reading *The Other Side of the Closet,* a book about the coming-out crisis for heterosexual spouses of gay and lesbian people, by Amity Pierce Buxton.

? Should gay parents hide their sexual orientation from their children?

See chapter 4, "Family and Children."

? Why do gay people have to be so public about it or "flaunt it"?

Several years back, my uncle said to me, "Okay, I can understand wanting to be truthful about who you are, but why do gays have to flaunt it all the time?" When he asked me that question, my uncle and I were sitting on beach chairs just a few feet away from the picnic table where my uncle's mother-in-law was playing Scrabble with my friends David and Irene, who were just a couple of months away from being married.

At that moment, David was stroking Irene's back in a very tender and loving way. I called my uncle's attention to the obvious public display of affection—David and Irene were clearly "flaunting" their heterosexuality—and asked my uncle if he considered what David was doing with Irene "flaunting." He got my point.

What we generally consider normal behavior for heterosexual people—talking about a romantic interest or relationship, an affectionate peck on the cheek between husband and wife, holding hands in public, or stroking the back of your beloved—we call "flaunting" when gay and lesbian people do it. (I've also heard people complain, "Why do they have to shove it down our throats!")

Most gay people, like heterosexual people, have no desire to make a spectacle of themselves. They just want to go about their lives in the same way that heterosexual people do. Many times I've heard lesbian and gay people say—and I've said it, too—how wonderful it would be to hold hands when walking down the street with a boyfriend, girlfriend, or spouse without fear of someone calling you names or coming after you with a baseball bat.

? What is National Coming Out Day?

National Coming Out Day, which has been celebrated every October 11 since 1988, commemorates the October 11,

1987, gay and lesbian rights march on Washington, D.C. The annual celebration is sponsored by the Human Rights Campaign (HRC), a national political organization that champions gay and lesbian rights issues.

National Coming Out Day is part of a visibility campaign that encourages "lesbian, gay and bisexual Americans to come out of the closet with pride every day." The idea behind National Coming Out Day is for gay people to tell the truth about their lives—to come out of the closet—in order to put to rest the myths that society has used against them.

National Coming Out Day is now marked by events in places all over the world. For more information, visit the Web site for HRC (www.hrc.org).

4

Family and Children

❓ Can gay people have families? What kinds of families do they have?

Besides their extended families (parents, siblings, aunts, uncles, and cousins), gay people have created their own families. For example, Leslie and Joanna and their infant daughter, Emily, are a family. David and Edward, who just celebrated their twenty-fifth anniversary, think of themselves as a family. Al, who divorced his wife because he is gay, and his two teenage sons who live with him full-time are a family. Evelyn, a retired math teacher, and three of her friends, all lesbians, who share a large home on Cape Cod, in Massachusetts, call themselves their "chosen family."

These families may not match the 1950s ideal of the nuclear family as portrayed in that era's television situation comedies, but no family can meet that fictional standard. What these families *do* have is what all families ought to have: love, care, concern, and commitment to the health, happiness, and well-being of each family member.

I like to think that heterosexuals could learn a few things from the families that gay people have worked so hard to create.

Is it true that gay people are antifamily or that they want to destroy traditional families?

No. Despite what some antigay activists have said and continue to claim, gay and lesbian people and gay rights organizations do not want to destroy traditional families, nor do they oppose family values—especially since most gay people share these same family values and value their place in the lives of their families.

What most gay and lesbian people *would* like is to be accepted by their families as full and equal members. They would like the definition of *family* to be broadened to include the realities of American family life—a reality that includes gay and lesbian families of all kinds. And they would like their couple relationships and their relationships with their children to be protected by law in the same way that those of heterosexuals are protected.

Do gay people want to be parents?

Like heterosexual people, many gay and lesbian people want to be parents, and for all the same reasons. For example, David and Kevin, who are both in their early thirties, knew they wanted to be parents even before they met. "I come from a large, happy family," said David. "Early on I saw the importance of being in a family environment. Since my nephew and niece were born and since many of my friends have had children, I've seen how emotionally rewarding it can be. And as I've gotten older, my paternal instincts have gotten very strong."

David and Kevin live in a state that allows gay couples to adopt jointly, so this is the route they've chosen. They hope to adopt privately in the United States, but if that doesn't work out, their plan is to adopt outside the county.

Do gay people have children? How? Can gay people and/or gay couples adopt?

Yes, gay people have children. For example, among the six hundred thousand same-gender couples identified in the 2000 U.S. census, one-third of the lesbian couples and one-fifth of the male couples had children in their households.

Some gay people have children from a prior heterosexual marriage. And others choose to have children in all the same ways that straight people do, with one exception. Same-gender couples cannot have biological children together—which means they can't accidentally conceive—so having a child generally requires considerable thought and effort.

Even with considerable thought and effort gay couples can't necessarily get joint legal custody of their children, because state adoption laws don't all make provisions for families where both parents are the same gender. In such a case only one parent is the legal parent; the other parent has no legal relationship with his or her child.

Some states explicitly prohibit gay people and gay couples from adopting altogether. In addition, when it comes to other methods of having children, including surrogacy and artificial insemination, state laws are inconsistent and can vary dramatically from one state to the next.

Fortunately for gay and lesbian people who wish to have children, there are extensive resources and experienced legal experts who can help. For state-by-state information on laws regarding adoption, donor insemination, surrogacy, and custody and visitation laws, I suggest that you visit the Web site for the Family Pride Coalition (www.familypride.org). The Human Rights Campaign also provides extensive information on this subject on its Web site (www.hrc.org).

? Why do some people object to gay men and lesbians being parents?

Here are some of the absurd arguments that are made by people who object to gay men and lesbians having, adopting, and raising children: gay parents are more likely to molest their children; gay parents will raise gay and lesbian children; children raised by two parents of the same gender will have psychological problems; the children of gay parents will be discriminated against. And finally, the fall-back argument that has been used to justify keeping kids in foster care rather than allowing them to be adopted by gay people: all children should have a mother and father.

First, gay and lesbian people are no more likely to sexually abuse their children than are heterosexual people. (And, as the Children's Hospital study I cite in chapter 1 suggests, gay and lesbian parents are far less likely to do so.) Second, you can't intentionally raise a gay child any more than you can intentionally raise a straight child. Third, whether a child is well adjusted has far more to do with whether the child is loved than with the gender or sexual orientation of the child's parent or parents. Every study that I've seen in recent years has concluded that the sexual orientation of the parent has no impact on a child's psychological well-being.

There's no question that kids with gay parents are likely to face challenges that straight kids don't, but that's a result of society's prejudice and not the parenting abilities of gay people. Because of prejudice and the potential for harassment, children of gay people may feel compelled to hide the fact that their parents are gay. If they choose not to hide the truth about their parents, they may have to contend with prejudiced remarks or negative reactions from other children and/or the parents of those children. But prejudice is not a reasonable justification for denying gay people the right to raise kids any more than it is for denying that right to any other group in society that experiences prejudice. It is, however, a great argument for working to change attitudes.

And finally, in a perfect world we would all be raised by at least two loving, stable parents, within a community made up of grandparents, aunts, uncles, family friends, and caring neighbors. With all due respect to my late parents, simply having a mother and a father is no guarantee that family life will be perfect or even happy.

? Do gay parents raise gay children?

Sure, gay people sometimes raise kids who are gay, and so do heterosexual parents. But that doesn't mean that gay parents make their kids gay or that heterosexual parents make their kids heterosexual. It simply means that all parents, straight and gay, wind up with a certain percentage of kids who are gay—and that percentage is apparently the same for gay parents as it is for straight parents.

Are lesbian couples better suited to raising children than male couples? Can't two women raise kids better than two men can? Isn't there a natural "mothering instinct" that two men don't have?

I interviewed an "expectant" male couple quite a few years back, when gay couples with children weren't nearly so common as they are today. The two men were in the delivery room with the woman who was giving birth to the child they were going to adopt. One of the attending nurses was calling out the baby's progress like an announcer at a football game. As the men described the scene, the nurse started with "Here he comes," progressed to "There's his head," and then, at last, "Here he is!" And the final comment was a shocked, "Oh my God, he's a *she!*"

No one knew the gender of the child in advance of its birth, but the nurse just assumed that two men had to be having a boy. The couple were delighted by the arrival of their daughter and amused by the surprise of the nurse. But they were less amused as they found themselves responding to questions from concerned adults—parents, friends, and complete strangers—about the abilities of two men to raise a girl. They never doubted their abilities to parent their child. And because they also want their daughter to have strong female role models, they've made a special effort to include in their lives close women friends and extended family.

Gender is not a deciding factor in one's ability to raise children, whether that child is a boy or a girl. Children seem to adapt and respond in their own ways to the circumstances of their family life. I'm reminded of another couple I interviewed, two men with a teenage daughter. I asked her what she called her two dads, and she said that one was her Daddy Daddy and the other was her Mommy Daddy. The funny thing was, the Mommy Daddy was an outwardly masculine, gruff kind of guy, and the Daddy Daddy was the softer, more stereotypically gay guy. But their outward appearance obviously had no bearing on the roles they played in their daughter's life, at least the way she interpreted those roles in comparison to her friends who had female mothers and male fathers.

? What happens when gay couples with kids split up? Who gets the kids? What if one parent dies?

Plenty of gay and lesbian couples, like heterosexual couples, split up. And when kids are involved it can be especially complicated, because for gay and lesbian couples who have children, often only one parent is the legal parent (adoptive or biological).

When gay and lesbian couples in this situation can agree on custody arrangements—which, ideally, they have put into writing prior to having the child or prior to their separation—there are no problems beyond the usual challenges divorced couples with children face. But when a gay or lesbian couple who have a child can't agree on custody arrangements, and only one parent is the legal parent, the other parent will likely find he or she has no legal rights.

For couples where both parents are legal parents—that is, both have legally adopted the child, or one is the biological parent and the other is a legal adoptive parent—there is plenty of legal precedent to be followed should the parents be unable to agree on custody arrangements.

In the event a parent dies, the surviving parent will retain custody of the child or children as long as that parent is the biological or legal adoptive parent. If the surviving partner is not the biological or legal adoptive parent, the outcome can be disastrous, because in the eyes of the law that parent has no legal relationship with the child. If the second parent wishes to gain custody of the child, he or she may face a difficult legal battle to gain custody, particularly if the child's legal next of kin wishes to assume custody.

? Should gay parents hide their sexual orientation from their children? Is there a right time to tell their kids?

Sometimes parents must keep their homosexuality a secret from their children out of necessity. For example, if a parent is leaving a heterosexual marriage and is embroiled in a custody battle in which his or her sexual orientation could affect the outcome, hiding the truth is essential.

For parents who are not faced with a custody battle like the one I've described, what they decide to do about disclosing their sexual orientation will depend on their specific circumstances and their personal preferences. For example, if an openly gay male or lesbian couple is raising a child together from infancy, it is extremely unlikely that they will hide the nature of their relationship from their child. The child will have observed her parents as a couple and will over time become aware that her parents are gay or lesbian, so the parents will have nothing to disclose.

For a parent who has left a heterosexual marriage, it's a matter of deciding whether to tell a child that his parent is something different from what he thought he was. If the gay or lesbian parent has custody of that child, it could be very difficult to hide the truth, especially if the parent is actively dating or has a new partner. Kids aren't stupid, and if there's a secret to be found out, they'll make every effort to uncover the truth. If, on the other hand, the parent does not have custody and the child visits only during designated times, it is easier to hide the truth.

There is a rule of thumb for parents who choose to come out to their children: the sooner the better. That was what Lloyd, the father of a teenage son and daughter, learned from other gay fathers he met through a local support group. "I found out that the younger the children, the easier it was," said Lloyd. "Especially before they were teens and dealing with their own sexuality and were more aware about sexual things and had peer pressure. When they're younger, they're more accepting of things. They're not even so sure what 'gay' is. They just want to know that their father is still their father."

Joy Schulenburg, a lesbian mom and the author of *Gay Parenting*, concurs that children deal better with the news that a parent is gay when they're still young: "Among the children I talked to and corresponded with, there were distinct differences in attitudes between those who had been under twelve when they learned their parent was gay and those who had been twelve and over.

"The under-twelve age group seemed largely indifferent to their parent's sexual orientation (which is true also of children of heterosexuals). Most of them simply didn't understand what all the fuss was about. Parents were loved because they were parents, despite any personal quirks and without reservations. Once puberty set in, with its sexual awakening and attending social pressures, reactions varied and the incidence of concern and initial rejection increased."

? How do kids react to gay parents?

How children react to a parent's sexual orientation depends to a large degree on when they find out a parent is gay. For a child who has been raised since birth or early childhood by two parents of the same gender, the awareness is evolutionary. At first the child may be aware only that she has two parents of the same gender who sleep in the same bed.

Eventually she will realize that her other friends have parents of the opposite gender and will likely ask her parents why she has two daddies or two mommies instead of a mommy and a daddy. Then she'll learn the words for what her parents are and gain a fuller understanding of what it all means. For a child like this, there is no one moment of revelation when she discovers that her supposedly heterosexual parent is gay. So for this child there is no real news to react to.

When children are raised by opposite-gender parents and later one of the parents discloses that he or she is gay, children react in a variety of ways, from shock and rejection, to relief that their parent has finally confirmed what they already knew, to plain indifference.

Tina, who has been a stepmother to her partner's two sons since they were preteens, concluded from her experience that the way children ultimately respond to their parents' homosexuality has a great deal to do with the kind of relationship the parents have with their children: "The secret really turns out to be, do you have a loving relationship with your kids? And if you love and respect them, they tend to love and respect you. It's something that needs a lot of attention and work and commitment, like any relationship."

Kids want the love and attention of their parents. They want parents who will listen to them, set boundaries, and help them make their way in the world. Sexual orientation has no bearing on the ability of people to provide these key things to their children.

Do children of gay parents have special problems?

The world is not always a very friendly place for gay and lesbian people, and that can make it a challenging place for their children as well.

Nonetheless, beyond the potential for teasing and ridicule from their peers, especially in adolescence, the kids of gay parents do not have special problems. All the studies I've read since the early 1990s have come to the same conclusion on this subject: there are no psychological disadvantages for children being raised by gay people in comparison to those raised by heterosexuals.

When kids have two moms or two dads, what do they call them?

What may be a perplexing dilemma for an adult who is trying to imagine how a child figures out what to call two mommies or two daddies has been no problem for the kids I've talked to.

Susan, who is ten, calls her fathers, who have raised her since birth, Papa Don and Daddy David. Michael, who is twenty-four, calls his natural father Dad and his father's partner, who raised him since he was nine, Mama Chuck. Ellen and Doug, who are in their twenties, call their mother Mom and their mother's partner, whom she's been with for the last ten years, by her first name.

Is there an organization for gay people who have children?

There are several around the country. One of the oldest is the Family Pride Coalition, an international organization that supports, educates, and advocates for gay, lesbian, bisexual, and transgender parents and their families. They maintain an extensive and informative Web site (www.familypride.org).

? What about an organization for people who have gay parents?

It's called Children of Lesbians and Gays Everywhere (COLAGE). Their Web address is www.colage.org.

5

For Parents of Gay Children

? How can parents tell if their child is gay or lesbian?

You may sense it. You may have a hunch. You may suspect it. You can make an educated guess based on hundreds of little things or just gut instinct. But you can't know with absolute certainty whether your child is gay or lesbian until that child tells you—or otherwise indicates their sexual orientation through action or words. That's because there are no definitive universal outward signs and most gay people look and act like everyone else.

What about the effeminate boy who likes to play with dolls? Good chance. But not every effeminate boy who likes to play with dolls winds up with same-gender sexual orientation. (And, of course, most gay men did not start life as effeminate children.) What about a girl who hates dresses, likes to play with trucks, is built like a mini-linebacker, and wants to be a boxer? Possibly. But how do you explain the young woman I had dinner with recently who was just like that as a child and now lives quite happily with her boyfriend (who likes to cook, enjoys reading books, and hates sports)?

It can be especially difficult for parents to tell if their child is gay or lesbian because gay and lesbian kids often work very hard to hide from their parents any possible outward sign—behavioral, verbal, or emotional—that they're gay. So it may be impossible to determine whether your child is struggling with his or her sexual orientation or is simply troubled by adolescent angst.

? If you think your eight-year-old son or daughter is gay, is that too young to tell?

It's not too young to consider it as a possibility or even to have a strong sense, especially in those children who exhibit some of the classic stereotyped outward signs that we associate with male or female homosexuals. As I write later in this chapter, that's the case with Lillian and her young son, Andrew, who she suspects is gay based on her observations and gut sense.

Lillian won't know for certain until Andrew is older, but based on her suspicions Lillian has made an effort to learn more about homosexuality, and she's keeping a careful eye on how Andrew is treated by his classmates at school. He's already been called names by some of the other kids—mostly "fag" and "gay"—something Andrew didn't hesitate to tell his mother. Lillian had expected she would need to advise Andrew on how to deal with the name-calling and was prepared to speak with his teacher and the principal, if necessary. But for now Andrew has handled things on his own—and rather impressively, from what Lillian has told me.

This is what happened: When one of Andrew's classmates called him "gay," Andrew marched up to the name-caller and said, "I bet you don't even know what *gay* means!" In fact, the name-caller did not and shrugged. Andrew explained that *gay* meant a boy who liked boys and a girl who liked girls. Then he scolded the name-caller and said, "If you're going use a word like that, you should know what you're talking about."

Not all kids have such strong egos, nor are all kids comfortable telling parents that they're being called names. When that happened to me at summer camp when I was in my midteens, I was terrified of telling even my counselor that I was being called a fag, because I was afraid that he would think I *was* a fag. I would have died before I told my mother, and in fact I didn't tell her about the camp incident until I was in my forties.

? What should you do if you think your child is gay?

If you think your child is gay and you are not yet an expert on the subject, become one. Because when the day comes that you and your child discuss his sexual orientation, you want to know what you're talking about. And if you do know what you're talking about, you'll be a hero in your child's eyes.

If it turns out that your child isn't gay, well, then you'll still be an expert, and you can count on using what you've learned to advise a friend or relative. As I've discovered over the years, virtually everyone knows someone gay, and virtually everyone needs help sorting things out, whether the sorting out involves your own child, a friend's child, a friend, a parent, or a grandparent. Or you'll simply be in a better position to argue gay rights issues on something other than pure emotion.

Should you ask?

Sometimes young people want to be asked, which was the case with me when I was in my late teens. I had been dropping hints to my mother, but I didn't think—consciously anyway—that I wanted her to ask me outright if I was gay. But over time I dropped enough hints that she asked. And I answered in the affirmative.

With younger kids, asking may be inappropriate, especially if the child is still working his or her way through puberty and is unclear about his or her feelings of sexual attraction. In any case, asking directly can be self-defeating. I know plenty of people who in response to a parent's point-blank inquiry answered no or said, "It's none of your business."

In general, I think the safer course of action is to find a way to let your child know that you are comfortable with gay people and gay issues. And there are various ways to do this, from discussing gay issues in the news in an affirmative manner over dinner, to providing your kids with age-appropriate gay-affirmative books, whether fiction or nonfiction, to simply avoiding dismissive or negative comments regarding gay people and gay issues.

For example, one mother e-mailed me about her concerns that the youngest of her four sons was gay. It wasn't something her ten-year-old son brought up, but she and her husband noticed that the three older boys were starting to make offhand remarks to their little brother. They had to admonish the older boys on several occasions when they called their younger brother a fag, as well as several times when they criticized something he'd done by saying, "Don't be so gay." It made them take notice and caused them to wonder if there was something their sons were picking up on that they hadn't.

The mother's instinct was not to say anything directly, in part because she wasn't sure whether her youngest was indeed gay or, if he was, that he was fully aware of his feelings at such a young age. But she wanted to be sure he knew that his parents had no problem with him being gay, if that was in fact his orientation. And they wanted to educate their three older sons about gay people without being ham-handed or drawing attention to the youngest son.

My suggestion to her, as it has been to many parents, whether they have young children or older children, was to talk to her kids about a book she had read that she thought they would be interested in reading and to just leave it around the house. The book I suggested is a version of this book that I wrote for children ages ten and up, called *What If Someone I Know Is Gay?* I even suggested to her that she say it was written by an acquaintance, so it didn't seem as if she was dropping it on them completely out of the blue. So she got a copy of the book and, when the time was right, mentioned it to her sons and then left it in the family room.

Over a period of days all the boys thumbed through the book. At their mother's instigation they talked briefly about the book one evening, but that was pretty much that. However, although there wasn't further discussion, she noticed that the three older boys no longer teased their younger brother. And in the three years since, she and her husband have not had to say another word to them about the teasing.

Is the youngest son gay? He's now in deep adolescence, and his parents are still not sure. But what the parents know is that if and when their son decides to confide in them, he will do so with the knowledge that his parents love him enough to have educated themselves and his brothers in anticipation of that day.

If it strikes you as appropriate to ask your child directly if he or she is gay, there are ways to go about it that are less direct and potentially less confrontational than simply asking, "Are you gay?" You can say, for example, "I have the sense that something may be upsetting you, and I wanted to let you know that if it concerns your sexual orientation, your mother and I love you and we're here for you if you would like to speak with us." Or you can say more directly, "I have the sense that you may be gay or lesbian, and if that's the case, please know that your father and I love you," and so forth.

This is also not something you have to figure out on your own. You can easily consult with a counselor who has experience in these matters, or you can contact a local chapter of Parents, Families and Friends of Lesbians and Gays (PFLAG)—their Web address is www.pflag.org—and talk to a parent who has been down this road and can advise you on how to handle your specific circumstances.

? Why is it such a big deal for gay people to come out to their parents?

See chapter 3, "Coming Out / Going Public."

? If your son or daughter comes out to you, what should you do/say?

When a child comes out to you, what they need from you is reassurance. So ideally you'll say, "We love you. We always have. We always will. Knowing that you're gay doesn't change that." A child may also welcome hearing "It must have been very difficult keeping this secret from us" or "We wish we had known sooner so that we could have been of help to you. How can we be of help to you now?"

There are things that are better left unsaid to a child who has just shared with you the truth about his or her sexual orientation. For example, don't talk about how devastated you are, or about your disappointment. Don't ask your child if he or she is sure; they wouldn't have told you if they weren't sure. And don't suggest that it's just a phase or something that can be cured.

This is one of those moments in your life as a parent when your child needs you to be a parent above all else, and that means first and foremost taking care of the needs of your child. You can deal with your own issues—disappointment, anxiety, upset, and so on—without involving your child. This isn't to say that you can't ask for help. Your child will likely help you learn what you need to know and may even recommend things for you to read. But that first discussion should be about your child, not you.

? What if they're preteen? How can they know?

Children generally have a sense of their feelings of attraction—and that goes for all kids, not just gay kids. Though these are not the fully developed feelings of sexual attraction that come to the fore during adolescence, they are still there. When I was a kid I had a sense of those feelings, just as other gay kids probably have—remember that crush in third grade?—but I had no word to attach to them. Gay issues and gay people were not subjects anyone talked about, and there certainly weren't prime-time television programs with identifiable gay characters.

Kids growing up today who have same-gender orientation now have a name for what they're feeling, and some have a pretty good understanding of what that means. And some of those children feel comfortable sharing their thoughts, concerns, or confusion about those feelings with their parents.

That was the case with Dean's ten-year-old son, Sean. One evening when Dean was putting his son to bed, Sean asked his father, "Dad, do you think I'm gay?" As Dean explained to me later, this was really not a possibility he'd considered before, although he'd always had a sense that Sean was different from most of the other boys his age. "I hadn't thought about it in terms of his sexual orientation, because he's a great athlete, but he's also a really sensitive kid emotionally, mostly in the best sense of that word. Maybe I'm a prisoner of the era in which I grew up, and I should have known better, but I figured if he was great at sports he couldn't be gay."

Dean is not new to the subject of homosexuality. He has gay friends and gay relatives, but this was not a conversation he expected to be having with his ten-year-old son, a son he adores. With his heart pounding, Dean took a deep breath and asked his son if he knew what it meant to be gay. Sean said he did and explained that it was when a boy marries another boy or a girl marries another girl.

Recognizing that Sean knew what he was talking about, Dean said, "I don't know if you're gay, and that's something you'll come to understand as you grow up. But I want you to know that your mother and I love you and we will love the person you decide to marry, whether that person is a young man or a young woman." With that, Dean's son kissed him good night, and at least one of the two of them had a restful night's sleep.

If I think my child is gay, or if my child has just come out to me, how can I get information that's useful to my family's specific circumstances?

No two families are alike, so no two situations are exactly alike. If you think your child is gay, or you've recently found out, you need to find the appropriate way to handle your specific circumstances. That means reading whatever useful material you can get your hands on—you'll find an extensive bibliography at the back of this book—and talking to other parents who have gay kids.

The best place to start is with Parents, Families and Friends of Lesbians and Gays (PFLAG). Visit their Web site (www.pflag.org) or call them (see the "Resources" section at the back of this book), review the material available there, locate a PFLAG chapter near you, and get in touch with parents who have already been down the road you are on. These parents can provide the kind of personal, specific advice you need.

When I first told my mother I was gay, she was clearly upset. I suggested she contact PFLAG. She suggested I see a psychiatrist. Like mother, like son. We both dug in our heels and did nothing. Fast-forward twenty years and my mother was chair of the New York City PFLAG chapter's annual awards dinner and I was seeing a great therapist. We could have saved ourselves a fair amount of misery if we'd taken each other's advice early on, but better late than never. Please don't follow our example.

What if you accidentally discover that your child is gay? Should you say anything?

I received an e-mail from a woman who sneaked a look at her son's personal journals and discovered that he was gay. She wanted to talk to him about it, especially since he seemed to be struggling with his feelings. She suspected from observing him that he was depressed—which was why she decided to have a look at his journals in the first place—and she feared that he might even be suicidal.

One can argue whether this woman did the right thing by invading her son's privacy, but I could easily understand why she did what she did. She was concerned about her son's well-being, and she had a genuine fear that he might do himself harm. For that reason I advised her to get her son to a counselor, one who had experience dealing in an affirmative way with gay people.

I also recommended that she not disclose to her son that she had learned from reading his journals that he was struggling with his sexuality. In this circumstance, I suggested, it would be best to tell her son that she had a sense he was depressed and that she wanted him to talk to someone about it. To tell him that she'd read his journals and learned from them that he was gay could prove explosive. There was nothing to be gained by sharing with her son knowledge of what he'd chosen not to share with her in the first place.

I've also heard from parents who have walked in on their child having sex with someone of the same gender, discovered hidden pornography, or found that their child had been looking at gay pornography online. In these cases there was more to deal with than just the discovery that a child was gay. My suggestion here is to take a deep breath, count to ten, and think before you act.

? How do parents react to learning that their child is gay?

The most encouraging change I've seen since I first started writing on this subject in 1986 is how much more parents know about homosexuality and how much more they're focused on their child's well-being than on their own disappointment, shock, embarrassment, or anger. I don't mean to suggest that this is universal. But years ago, almost without exception, when I heard from parents who had just discovered that a child was gay, they were most likely to be focused on themselves and what the neighbors would think.

In recent years, I'm more likely to hear from parents—who may or may not be upset by what they've just learned—whose primary concern is how they can be supportive of their child and protect them from a world that they know is not always welcoming of gay people. This is especially true of parents who have preteens or adolescents they suspect or know are gay.

In general, how parents react to the news that a child is gay has a lot to do with who the parents are: the communities they come from, their ethnic or racial backgrounds, whether or not they are deeply religious, their familiarity with gay people, and so forth. And, in general, no matter how open-minded parents are—even if half their friends are gay or they already have one gay child or they are actively involved in working for gay rights—they are likely to be upset by the news that a child is gay. They may be upset for themselves or they may be upset for their child or both. So parents are likely to have a range of reactions.

To give you an idea of the different ways in which parents react, I thought I'd offer a few samples from my files:

Andrea's Parents

Many parents, although upset by the news that a child is gay or lesbian, manage to deal in a loving way with their child. Andrea's mother and father responded with tears. "They weren't the only ones crying," said Andrea, who said she is now closer to her parents than before she came out to them. "There was a lot I didn't understand, and I know this isn't what they wanted for me, but as much as they were hurting, they managed to tell me that I was their daughter and they loved me. There are still times when it isn't easy. Like the first time I brought my girlfriend home for dinner, they were really nervous. But, then, Penny and I were really nervous, too."

Lillian

Andrew's mother had a sense very early in her son's life that he was gay. "There was something about him," Lillian said, "his ease with his girlfriends, his manner, how he liked to curl up in a corner with a book. I wondered. And then we were at the grocery one day when he was nine. The cashier was this extremely cute teenage boy, and the look Andrew had in his eyes. . . . I don't know quite how to describe it, but it was a look that had such meaning. This wasn't hero worship. I've seen that. This was different. It was like an electric charge was going through him. I just knew."

The first thing Lillian did when she was alone after the visit to the grocery store was to go to her bedroom and cry. "I felt so silly, especially because he was so young. But I could picture the future ahead of him, and we've all seen how cruel children can be. And that's what made me so sad."

Beyond her sadness, Lillian was confused. Was she really right? What, if anything, should she say to Andrew? Should she talk to her husband?

Lillian decided to talk to her husband, and they agreed that they would do whatever was necessary to make certain their son had a good life. The biggest challenge for them was finding information on how to raise a great gay kid. It was around this time that Lillian wound up sitting next to me on a flight to New Orleans. (See the introduction to this book for that story.)

Karen

When Karen learned that her twenty-seven-year-old son, Alex, was gay, she had no reassuring words for him, because her tears were not about him. Karen, a junior high school teacher, was crying because she felt betrayed and was furious. She recalled, "I wanted him dead, and I told him so."

To Karen, the son she had known died in that moment of revelation, and she was not at all happy with her "new" son. And she was terrified of anyone finding out.

What is often hardest for parents like Karen to cope with is a sense of embarrassment and/or fear of what friends, neighbors, relatives, or even strangers will think if they find out. Paradoxically, while the gay child who comes out of the closet is now free of the burden of hiding the truth, parents of gay children may then find themselves in a closet of their own, hiding the truth about their child. Every time they're faced with a question like "Is your son married?" or "Is your daughter dating anyone?" parents have to decide what to say.

In the first years after Alex came out to Karen—and well after she begged Alex to forgive her for what she had said, which he did—Karen told a handful of her colleagues about her gay son. And they were all supportive. But she's still having a difficult time. "Hardly a day goes by when one of the other teachers doesn't come bouncing into school talking about a new grandchild," she said. " 'Don't worry, this will happen to you soon,' they tell me. I used to run out to the bathroom and cry. Others say, 'The worst thing that could happen would be if my child were a homosexual.'

"I don't want their pity or rejection. I know I shouldn't feel this way. I should grow up, but that's how I feel. And I'm terrified of having my students find out. Almost every day they call each other 'fag.' Of course I feel compelled to scold them. If only they knew."

My Mom

It was not easy for my mom at first, but there was an incident that occurred about ten years after I first told her I was gay that was a major turning point for her. She told me, "When your first book [*The Male Couple's Guide*] was published, I brought it to a family dinner. I can't remember why you weren't there.

"I was very proud of you and wanted to show the book to those who were present. I started to speak about the book, but before I said what it was about, some relatives at the table asked to see it, and when it came into their hands, they looked at it, never said a word, and changed the subject. It was as if someone smacked me in the face. I realized that for some people it wasn't even a subject to be spoken about.

"After that," she said in a conversation with me some years after the incident, "I refused to hide you. If I spoke about my children I had to speak about all my children, their lives, the fact that two were married, and that one was gay and in a relationship. Otherwise I would be ashamed of myself for hiding."

My mom had this final word for parents with gay kids: "Parents who are still ashamed of their gay and lesbian children need to look at why they're not questioning what they've been told by society. Most of our children are healthy, decent, caring, sensitive people, and we fail them when we join the rest of society in denying who they are. We are their parents. If we don't defend their right to live full lives, who will?"

? If your child is gay, does that mean you did something wrong as a parent?

No.

? If your young child tells you he or she is gay, does that mean your child was sexually abused?

No, but it's certainly an opportunity to have an age-appropriate discussion about sexuality.

? If one of your children is gay, is there a greater chance that one of your other children will be gay, too?

There's been no conclusive research on this, but anecdotally, and from what I've seen, it's not uncommon in families where one child is gay for a second child to be gay as well.

? What's it like for parents who have two or more gay kids?

For parents who have dealt in a constructive way with the news that a child is gay, the news that a second child is gay is likely to be dealt with in a constructive way as well. And because such parents have experience with one gay child, the territory will be far more familiar—and easier, one hopes—the second time around. Needless to say, the opposite is true as well, and in that case a second gay child may only deepen the upset.

In that vein, I remember a heartbreaking story told to me several years ago by friends who owned a gay bookstore in Denver. They lived in an apartment above their store and were awakened by a woman banging on the store's front door at 7:00 a.m. They recalled: "She was wearing a pink quilted bathrobe, pink fluffy slippers, and had pink curlers in her hair. At first we thought she was angry about something, but when we opened the door we could see she'd been crying. She explained that the day before she had learned that two of her six children—three boys and three girls—were gay. She'd already known about the one, and then a second son came out to her.

"Early that morning, she called her eldest daughter in New York to tell her the news, and her daughter, who was happily married with children of her own, said, 'Oh, mother, how could you be so blind? I'm the only straight one. They're all gay!' Well, with that she started bawling, 'He's going to kill my babies, he's going to kill my babies!' It turns out her husband was very unhappy about the first gay child, and she was terrified of what would happen when he learned about the others.

"Well, we loaded her up with books and suggested she get in touch with the local PFLAG chapter and asked her to let us know how things turned out, but we never heard from her again."

One more story: Julie, who has three sons, two of them gay, discovered that it was Daniel, her youngest son, who had the problem, not her. "I already knew that Daniel was gay, but it was clearly something he didn't want to talk about. He had to know it wouldn't be a problem for me—I adore his brother and his brother's partner—but as I learned later, he felt bad about what this might mean to me.

"I remember Daniel's exact words when he explained to me why he waited until he was thirty—which was years after his brother came out—to speak with me about the fact that he was gay. He said, 'I couldn't imagine doing this to you.' As if he did anything to me! Frankly, it was a relief to consider the possibility of another son-in-law. My daughter-in-law and I work very hard at getting along, but it's never been a natural fit. Maybe it's my fault, but I seem to get along better with men."

? Do mothers and fathers react differently?

Mothers and fathers may react differently to a gay or lesbian child, but not consistently enough to generalize that fathers always have more trouble with their gay sons or that mothers always have more trouble with their lesbian daughters.

It's safe to say, however, that mothers and fathers often have different expectations for their children depending upon whether that child is a boy or a girl, and that their reactions to a child's homosexuality may be tied to these differing expectations.

For example, one father I spoke with who has two gay sons said, "Fathers train males to be macho, so being a 'he-man' is a very important thing. Fathers may expect to live their lack of success in that area through their children. I think with a gay son you may find more disappointment from the father at first. I don't think you find that as much in a mother."

? What if you're okay with the fact that your child is gay, but your spouse is not? How can you resolve the conflict?

I've heard from parents in this circumstance, and it can be extremely painful, difficult, and divisive both for the couple and for the family.

I suggest first speaking with other parents who have been through this experience by contacting your local chapter of Parents, Families and Friends of Lesbians and Gays (PFLAG) through their Web site (www.pflag.org). You can also try on your own to speak with and educate the spouse who is having a difficult time, but you may not find your efforts welcome. In such a case I suggest seeking professional counseling, and if your spouse won't go with you, I suggest going on your own.

? What if your child comes out to you but doesn't want you to tell the other parent? Should you keep it a secret?

There may be very legitimate reasons for not sharing this secret with a spouse. And generally it concerns the child's fear (or the parent's fear) that the other parent will react poorly—or even violently. If the child's concern is legitimate, you'll likely know it and for that reason won't hesitate to honor your child's wishes.

However, sometimes a child asks for the secret to be kept because the child is closer to one parent than the other, has simply misjudged his other parent, or perhaps hopes that the first parent will smooth the way with the second. It's impossible to make a general recommendation here, but for anyone contemplating asking a parent to keep such a secret, consider the potentially awkward position you're putting your parent in, especially if your parents have a close relationship. And secrets have a way of seeping out.

No two stories are alike, but here's one example where the secrets got a little complicated: Paulette Goodman discovered that her teenage daughter was gay in a letter she received from her daughter's ex-boyfriend. Goodman recalled, "In his letter he told me about my daughter's new friend and that he thought it was more than a friendship. I didn't breathe a word of this to my husband. I was afraid of how he would react."

In the months that followed, Goodman's daughter didn't say a word, although Goodman recalled late-night phone calls during her daughter's visits home. "I knew there was something going on, but I couldn't talk to her about it," she said. And while Goodman's daughter never said anything to her, Goodman decided to tell her husband about the letter. His response was a simple "So what?" "I was so relieved," Goodman said.

Three months later, Goodman's daughter came home for summer vacation. "She asked her dad to go for a ride with her," Goodman recalled, "and I realized that she was going to come out to him. When they came home, I was furious because I felt she didn't trust me. I was hurt. I'm her mother. I love her. I've always been crazy about her, yet for many years we had been on different planes. She was secretive. She was undergoing all kinds of things, a good part of which was dealing with her sexuality. And she was angry at me for some reason.

"So I confronted her, and we started to talk. She was crying. She said the only reason she didn't tell me was that she thought I'd never understand. She was afraid I wouldn't let her finish school, and that we would cut her off. She had heard terrible stories from other kids."

In a very short time, the Goodman family sorted things out and Paulette Goodman went on to become actively involved with her local PFLAG chapter and was ultimately elected national president of the organization.

? How do you talk to your child about sexually transmitted diseases, including HIV/AIDS, if they're gay? Is there anything special a parent should know?

It goes without saying that all parents need to discuss with their children, no matter what their sexual orientation, the importance of responsible sexual behavior, the dangers of sexually transmitted diseases, including HIV/AIDS, and how to protect oneself from infection.

Because HIV/AIDS is a disproportionately larger problem among gay men than it is among heterosexual men in the United States, it is perfectly legitimate for parents of sexually active gay males to be especially concerned. This is not a reason to impose your fears on your child, but it is a good reason to do your own research and to help educate your child about both the dangers posed by sexually transmitted diseases and the proven methods of prevention. (For more information on this subject, see the questions in chapter 7, "Sex", where I discuss this issue. Also see the "Resources" section at the back of this book for where to find detailed information on HIV/AIDS and other sexually transmitted diseases.)

? What should you do if your child is getting teased or harassed at school for being gay (or because they are perceived to be gay)?

The first thing to do when your child reports to you that they're being teased, harassed, or abused is to reassure your child that you love him or her and will do whatever is necessary to make sure they're safe. Because your child may fear that your involvement will make things worse by bringing more unwanted attention, he may argue with you about taking action. As a parent, you know what you have to do, so you will have to explain to your child that he deserves better, that the harassment is unacceptable, and that you'll be there to support him every step of the way.

Another concern your child is likely to have is that you'll think he or she is gay because of the nature of the teasing. So don't ask, "Well, are you gay?" Save that discussion for another time. Whether your child is gay is not the point. The point is that, whether they're gay or straight, they're being harassed. And that's the immediate problem.

The first thing to do, assuming there isn't reason to call the police, is to contact the school authorities. If it were my child, I'd start with the principal. If I didn't get satisfaction there, I would go to my local school board. There are also other resources you can call on for advice, from local antigay-violence organizations and gay legal defense groups to the Gay, Lesbian and Straight Education Network (GLSEN). See the "Resources" section at the back of this book for more information.

Not all children tell their parents they're being teased, harassed, or physically abused. And the likely reason for this is their fear of telling their parents *why* they're being teased. For example, Keith, who is now in college and comfortable being openly gay, was routinely teased, threatened, and on occasion beaten up from almost his first day of high school. "It was a good day if I got called 'fag' or 'gay' fewer than a dozen times," he said. "Sometimes I got tripped. Kids wrote things on my locker. And every now and then I'd get cornered on the school bus by some of the bigger boys and they'd punch and kick me. I wanted to tell my parents what was going on, but I was scared they would think I was gay if they knew the reason I was having trouble. And if they found out I was gay I figured I'd be even worse off."

Keith misjudged his parents, because in his senior year when he wound up with a broken nose, his parents demanded to know what had happened. "I was tired of hiding the truth," Keith said. "And I was so upset and scared that I broke down and told them everything. My parents were great, and boy, were they mad, but not at me. Still, I begged them not to say anything, but they went to the principal, demanded that she do something to make sure I was protected, and they called the police and had my chief tormentor arrested. It wasn't like I was never called 'fag' again, but it was only one or two kids, and they said it under their breath. It felt really good to know that if I had a problem I could go to the principal and that my parents were behind me 100 percent."

? How do I talk to other parents about my gay child?

How would you like other parents to respond to you? Are you looking for pity? Sympathy? Indifference? Respect?

No one says you have to say anything, although you may find this choice to be a difficult one to live by, especially if your child is of an age where his or her peers are settling down and getting married. You may find yourself having to remain silent while other parents exchange stories about their children and the lives they're leading. And if you're tempted to invent a life for your child that you think will be more acceptable for public consumption, resist the impulse. You don't want to get caught in a lie, especially if your child is the one who catches you.

If you choose to speak about your child in an honest and matter-of-fact way, and would like other people to respond to you in a respectful and matter-of-fact way, you've got to indicate to them in what you say that this is how you would like to be treated.

For example, when my mom traveled and found herself in conversations with people she had just met, and when the discussion worked its way around to children and grandchildren, she would say that she had three children, two sons and a daughter; that one son and one daughter were married; and that her older son had a partner. If there were puzzled looks and my mother was feeling politically frisky, she might say, "My older son and his partner would be married, but as you know gay people aren't allowed to legally marry, at least not yet."

? What should you say to the grandparents?

"Whatever you do, don't tell the grandparents!" "They're old. They'll never understand. They don't need to know. Let them die in peace. You're their favorite. Why destroy their image of you?" These are the kinds of exhortations from well-meaning family members (including one of my own) that many gay and lesbian people confront when they bring up the possibility of sharing the truth about their lives with the grandparents.

Grandparents are likely tougher than you think. Though they may greet the news of a gay grandchild with surprise, grandparents often prove more resilient and more accepting than parents, for all the same reasons that grandparents are almost always more accepting of what their grandchildren do than of what their own children do.

Bob and Elaine, who were active members of their local PFLAG chapter at the time I interviewed them in the late 1980s, told me my favorite story involving grandparents. Bob waited until a couple of years after his son came out to talk with his own parents—the grandparents—about his son's homosexuality.

This is what he told me: "I went to visit them and told them I had something to talk to them about. My mother asked if there was anything wrong, and I told her there was nothing wrong, but there was something I wanted to explain. So I said, 'You know all those Sundays when you wanted to come visit or you wanted Elaine and me to come here, and I said I had business appointments? We never had business appointments. Elaine and I are members of an organization, and we go to meetings. The organization is for parents of gays.'

"I stopped at that point, but they didn't react. So I asked, 'Do you know what "gay" is, Mom?' And my mother said, 'Sure, that's when a guy likes a guy.' And I added, 'Yeah, and when a girl likes a girl.' 'Oh,' she said, 'the girls do it, too?'

"So I proceeded to explain homosexuality, and I said, 'The reason we go to the meetings is that one of our sons is gay.' My mother said, 'Oh, we've known that for a long time.' My mouth fell open in awe. So I asked her which of my sons they thought was gay. And they said Jonathan. I said, 'You're right, but what made you think Jonathan was gay?' 'Well,' my mother said, 'when he talks his voice squeaks, and he uses his hands a lot when he talks.' I said, 'Mom, that has nothing to do with being gay.' I explained a bit more, and at some point they commented, 'They're entitled to do everything in life just like everyone else'."

Not all grandparents are that matter-of-fact, but it's important to remember that grandparents are not nearly as fragile, uninformed, or unwilling to learn new things as we may think.

My own grandmother proved to be extremely resilient, despite an initial round of crying that lasted about three days.

My family was not keen on me telling her, but my increasingly public career made it likely she'd find out anyway, and I didn't want her finding out from someone else. And most important to me was my need to know that my grandmother would still love me if she knew the truth about my life. Also, we'd always been very close, but because I'd not shared with her this key piece of information there was less and less we could talk about; both my work and my relationship life were off-limits. So, against my family's wishes, I told her.

One of the great joys in my life was the pleasure my grandmother took in being a part of the life that my partner and I had created. A very short time after meeting him, she began calling him her grandson, and he took to her like his own grandmother.

During the final years of my grandmother's very long life we had fun adventures together, from walks to the ocean, with both of us on either side of her as we negotiated the sandy Long Island beach, to birthday weekends at her favorite hotel in New York City. And along the way she became an outspoken defender of gay rights, accompanying me on occasion to speaking engagements, never missing a book signing or party right on through her ninety-ninth year. We both would have missed so much if I'd decided to "protect" her from the truth.

? What should you tell a child who has a gay aunt or uncle? How old do they have to be? How do nieces and nephews react?

What you say and how much you explain depends on the age of the child and the circumstances. Quite often children won't say anything, particularly if they've grown up with their uncle and his partner or aunt and her partner as a fact of life. But when kids start to recognize that not everyone has two cohabiting uncles or two cohabiting aunts, they're likely to ask their parents a question or two, like "Do the uncles sleep together?" "Are they married?"

Questions like these are easy to answer: "Yes, your uncles are a couple like your father and me, and they sleep together because they love each other." If the uncles are married, all you have to say is yes, and then be prepared for a follow-up comment like "I didn't know that two boys could get married." Of if they're not married, you have to decide how much you would like to explain. For example: "No, they're not married. They would like to be, but it's not legal for two men to marry in our state." And then be prepared for the inevitable and perfectly reasonable next question: "Why?"

For David and Kevin, who have been together since before David's niece and nephew were born, the nature of their relationship has never been an issue. "From the time they could speak," said David, "they called us Uncle David and Uncle Kevin. To them it seemed like the most natural thing in the world. I'm sure when they get older they'll have some questions about their two uncles. I've already talked with my brother and sister-in-law about this, so they'll know how to handle the questions. I think the real problems may come up when they start hearing things about 'fags' at school. But we'll deal with that when the time comes."

Because of my work, I thought I had done everything right in advising my brother and sister on how to explain things to my niece and nephews when the inevitable questions arose. But it turns out, much to my surprise, that I hadn't. I wrote a magazine essay about what happened, which you can find on my Web site (www.ericmarcus.com).

? Are there any organizations/groups for parents of gay people? What about parents of gay teenagers or preteens?

Parents, Families and Friends of Gays and Lesbians (PFLAG) is the gold standard, which is why I've cited the organization several times in this chapter. Founded in New York City in the early 1970s by Jeanne Manford and her gay son Morty (you can read about them in my book *Making Gay History*), PFLAG now has hundreds of chapters and affiliates across North America and a handful around the world. For complete contact information, see the "Resources" section at the end of this book.

6

Dating, Relationships, and Marriage

? How do gay people meet?

In the 1950s, when Barbara Gittings—a clerk-typist from Philadelphia who was later one of the pioneers of the gay rights movement—was a young woman, she desperately wanted to meet other women who were gay. The problem was, she'd only read about lesbians in novels. Through her reading, Gittings also learned the name of a gay bar in New York City, so she hitchhiked to New York and made her way to the bar. "When I finally found the place and found my people, it was marvelous," she recalled. "I don't like bars, but I was thrilled to meet people who were like me."

Though bars were just about the only places gay men and lesbians could go in the 1950s to meet other people like themselves, today in every major and midsize city, gay and lesbian people can meet in a variety of settings, from gay and lesbian running clubs and softball teams to religious organizations and volunteer groups—in addition to bars, restaurants, and clubs that cater specifically to a gay and lesbian clientele. Many cities also have gay and lesbian community centers, where various organizations meet and events of all kinds are held.

Gay people also meet in all the usual ways that all people meet: at work, at social events, at the grocery store, online, and through friends and family. When I was in my early twenties, for example, my mother and her friend Fran decided that their gay sons should meet. They figured that if they weren't going to have daughters-in-law of any kind, they might as well try for Jewish sons-in-law. It was a nice try.

? How do gay people recognize each other?

There's a secret dress code that only gay people know. In the old days gay men wore green ties and lesbians wore special pins. Today the dress code is more subtle, and we're all notified by e-mail on a monthly basis on the latest code update.

Had you going there for a second, didn't I?

Sometimes it's relatively easy for gay people to tell if the person they've just met is also gay. For example, if you meet at a gay church group, you can figure that just about everyone you meet there is gay. Or if you're in a nongay setting, and the person is wearing a button or jewelry that indicates support for gay causes, they're probably gay.

Another clue might be if the person's style of clothing conforms to what's popular among gay people. But the way a lot of teenagers dress these days, I sometimes think they're *all* gay! A lot of them have adopted fashions and hairstyles (not to mention the piercings and tattoos) that were once the exclusive domain of gay people.

But if there are no outward signs or the signs are inconclusive, it can be a major challenge. Some gay people talk about having "gaydar," which is sort of a sixth sense that a lot of gay people develop over time. It's an automatic gathering of evidence—clothes, manner, eye contact, verbal information—that may or may not lead you to conclude that the cute guy at work or that sexy female teaching assistant is gay. Gaydar, however, is far from infallible and is on occasion confused with wishful thinking.

Sometimes it can take days or weeks or more to get to know a person well enough to determine their sexual orientation or for them to feel comfortable enough to reveal it.

Here's just one story from a couple I interviewed for my long-term couples book, *Together Forever,* and their experience of figuring things out. When Jane met Justine in the company cafeteria, it was love at first sight, but Jane had no idea whether Justine was gay. She had her hopes, especially when Justine gave her a broad smile when they met, but she couldn't be sure.

Over the next couple of weeks, Jane gathered evidence from their conversations: "I found out that Justine lived alone. She never talked about boyfriends. Her politics seemed on-target. But it wasn't until I met her at her apartment one evening to go to the movies that I was absolutely sure. Her books were a dead giveaway."

Of course, Justine was also gathering evidence, so by the time she invited Jane to meet at her apartment before the movie, she was confident that Jane was also gay: "I could tell from the way she looked at me. Jane may have thought she was being subtle, but if there's one thing Jane isn't, it's subtle!"

? What do gay people do on a date?

Whether it's the first date or the tenth, what gay people do on a date varies as much as what heterosexual people do on dates. But because most gay people don't feel as comfortable—or as safe—being physical in public, you're far less likely to find gay people on dates holding hands across the dinner table at a restaurant or making out on the street, especially in suburban or rural areas.

? With two guys or two girls, how do you decide who makes the first move, who drives, who pays?

The more masculine one always pays, no matter the gender.

That's not true, but I know that that's what some people think. When you're two women or two men in a dating situation, it's difficult to fall into the standard boy-girl roles, unless you're both comfortable choosing compatible roles. For most gay and lesbian people, who makes the first move, who drives, who pays for the date, who makes the first call, and so forth are dictated by many different factors that are often not nearly as simple and clear-cut as the standard boy-girl routine that straight people can choose to follow.

So who pays for dinner may depend upon who asked whom out for the date or who makes more money. Or you may agree up front that you always split the costs. The one who reaches across the table to plant the first kiss may simply be the one who is feeling more confident at a given moment. And the one who drives may be the one who prefers to drive. While some people may see this lack of clearly defined roles as a challenge, I think it's an opportunity for people to figure out their likes and dislikes without being saddled with expectations based on gender.

? What should you do if you're straight and you think the person you're dating is gay?

If you think your boyfriend or girlfriend is gay, you can try asking them, "Are you gay?" But this may not work. If my first (and only) girlfriend in college had asked me if I was gay, I would have said no—not because I was trying to hide anything, but mostly because I still had so much trouble at that age even admitting it to myself. I learned years later from her that she suspected I was gay because of my lack of interest in doing anything physical other than kissing.

If you can't get what you feel is an honest response from the man or woman you're dating, you may find that your only alternative is to end the dating relationship. That doesn't mean you can't be friends, but there is no reason to subject yourself to a relationship with someone who would really rather be with a person of the same gender.

? What should you do if a gay person makes a pass at you?

If a gay person makes a pass at you and you're not interested, all you have to do is say some version of "Thanks, but I'm not interested." If a gay person makes a pass at you and you're interested, well then, this is your lucky day.

? Do gay people have long-lasting couple relationships?

Yes, and these relationships are full of all the joy, excitement, challenge, and satisfaction, as well as the hurt, disappointment, and tragedy, that straight people experience in their relationships.

There are no accurate statistics on the number of gay and lesbian couples (although about six hundred thousand chose to identify themselves in the 2000 U.S. census), but I can tell you from the research I've done and from anecdotal evidence that there are many gay and lesbian couples who have been together for ten, twenty, thirty, or forty years or more. And most of these couples have managed to do so in a culture that has been less than supportive of, and often hostile to, gay people and gay relationships.

? Are there more gay and lesbian couples than in years past? If so, why?

Yes, probably many more. There are several reasons for this, including changing societal attitudes toward gay people, changing expectations among gay people, changing expectations among our families, and more varied opportunities to meet potential partners.

When I wrote my first book, *The Male Couple's Guide*, which was published in 1988, the prevailing myth about gay and lesbian relationships was that they couldn't possibly last. Even though old myths die hard, most gay and lesbian people now know that satisfying, long-lasting relationships between gay partners are a reality, and those gay people who wish to have such a relationship actively pursue that possibility.

Finding a potential partner is now easier than it was in the past. First, there are more and more openly gay and lesbian people out there to choose from. Second, there are many more places and ways in which to meet.

Many gay couples can now also count on the kind of familial, religious, social, and even legal support that straight couples take for granted. For cxample, when Brent and Tom gave themselves a party for their tenth anniversary, Brent's parents and sister were an important part of the celebration. "Both sets of parents are very supportive of our relationship," said Brent. "Tom's parents would have been there, but they're a bit older than my parents, and the trip was just too much for them. But they called and sent a gift."

Tom and Brent have also formalized their relationship with a commitment ceremony at their local church and with a domestic partnership certificate offered by the city of San Francisco to unmarried couples. And when San Francisco briefly issued marriage certificates to gay couples in 2004, Tom and Brent were among the thousands of couples who waited in the rain for hours for the opportunity to legally marry. (For more on commitment ceremonies, domestic partnerships, and legal marriage, see the questions on these topics later in this chapter)

? Who plays the husband and who plays the wife?

When it comes to gay and lesbian relationships, this is the question I've been asked more than any other (although less frequently now than in the past). And I've been asked this question by people who are in traditional husband-wife relationships and by married professionals who have never assumed gender-defined roles.

For men and women in gay and lesbian couple relationships, decision-making, the division of labor, and who works or doesn't work (or who earns more or less) have nothing to do with defined husband-wife gender roles (how could they?) and nothing to do with who is more masculine or feminine. For example, who makes dinner is far more dependent on who gets home from work first than on who is more feminine. And decision-making depends on the individual personalities of the people in the relationship.

Like many heterosexual couples, some gay and lesbian couples follow a more traditional husband-wife model. For example, during the first year after male couple friends of mine adopted an infant girl, one stayed home taking care of the baby and did all the shopping, cleaning, and cooking. The other partner went to the office and provided the financial support for the whole family. The next year, they switched roles. Fortunately for them, their jobs permitted that kind of flexibility.

For another couple I met, both women had full-time jobs, but one partner performed the traditionally "female" chores, like cleaning the house and cooking, while the other partner took care of the traditional "male" chores, such as mowing the lawn, maintaining the car, and taking out the garbage. (As one of the women explained to me, "You don't need a penis to take out the garbage.") It just so happened that the more outwardly feminine of the two was the one who took care of the traditionally "male" chores.

? Who brings home the flowers? Who makes plans to celebrate Valentine's Day? Who drives?

Even among my most nontraditional straight couple friends, including couples in which the wives have profoundly successful careers, it's the husbands who bring their wives flowers, the husbands who plan something special for Valentine's Day (or risk being flogged), and the husbands who almost always drive the car.

With gay men and lesbians who are in couple relationships, unless they assume well-defined husband-wife routines, there is no falling back on traditional gender roles to figure out who should be giving whom the flowers and who should be seated behind the wheel. It just depends on individual expectations and preferences. When those expectations and preferences conflict, there can be plenty to work out.

For Joel and Tony, who have been together for nine years, their expectations about Valentine's Day, at least, coincide. Both think it's an important holiday to celebrate, so every year they've thought up surprises for each other. "The first year," explained Tony, "I got home from work early and made a trail of rose petals from the front door to the bedroom. So when Joel got home, he followed the trail, and I was there waiting for him. The candles were set out, I had our favorite music playing—you know, the whole nine yards."

Tony, of course, hadn't forgotten about the holiday either, and surprised Joel with a dozen yellow tulips and a bottle of his favorite wine. "I had also made reservations at our favorite restaurant," Tony told me. And what about driving? "I hate to drive, but I'm great at reading maps," said Tony. "And Joel loves to drive, but he never knows where he's going. So it works out well for us."

? Who plays the husband and who plays the wife in bed?

It simply depends upon who likes to wear the apron.

Oh, you'd like a serious answer.

For some gay and lesbian couples, one partner routinely takes the passive (or what some people might consider the traditional wife's) role and one partner takes the aggressive (or what some people might consider the traditional husband's) role. However, for most gay and lesbian couples—and, I suspect, most heterosexual couples as well—bedroom sexual habits aren't nearly so regimented. For more information on this subject, see chapter 7, "Sex."

? What are "butch-femme" relationships?

According to Lillian Faderman, as she writes about the butch-femme lesbian subculture in her book *Odd Girls and Twilight Lovers,* some lesbians, primarily young, working-class lesbians during the 1950s and 1960s, assumed either masculine ("butch") or feminine ("femme") roles. They expressed these roles in their manner of dress, demeanor, sexual behavior, and choice of partner: butches sought femmes, and femmes hoped to attract butches.

Today, while some lesbian couples and some gay male couples may play traditionally masculine and feminine roles, the strict butch-femme role-playing of earlier decades is no longer common.

? Are gay couples monogamous?

Is this anyone's business? I don't think so, but this is something my straight male friends, in particular, are curious—and misinformed—about, so I know I can't get away with skipping this question.

The common stereotype about gay male couples is that

they're not monogamous. As one of my heterosexual male friends said to me, "You're two guys. Without the civilizing influence of a woman, you can do what you want." Yeah, right. But what straight men fail to consider is how they would feel about being in a relationship where their partner was as free to have sex with other people as they were.

The issue of monogamy is complicated. For heterosexual married couples the general assumption is—and societal custom dictates—that they'll be monogamous, whether or not their marriage vows include a commitment to fidelity. What couples and individuals do in the privacy of their relationships is another matter entirely.

For gay male and lesbian couples, the rules regarding monogamy are the rules we make. Gay people in couple relationships may make assumptions based on their own personal beliefs, may have explicit conversations about what suits them best, and may argue about their differing expectations. And when agreed-upon rules are broken, they suffer all the hurt and disillusionment that heterosexuals do.

What I found in the forty interviews I did for my book on happy, long-lasting gay and lesbian relationships—hardly a scientific study—was that monogamy was an issue that just about all the couples had discussed, usually early in the relationship. All the lesbian couples I interviewed had chosen a "monogamous lifestyle," although that wasn't because they all agreed it was what they wanted. For these couples, monogamy proved to be what was best for the relationship.

Among the men I interviewed, the majority had committed to a monogamous lifestyle, but some had chosen a non-monogamous lifestyle. (And some who had been monogamous at the start of the relationship chose not to be later on and vice versa.) I hasten to add that a nonmonogamous lifestyle is not a relationship without rules. The couples I interviewed who led nonmonogamous lifestyles generally had very explicit rules about what was and was not permitted regarding sexual relations outside of the relationship.

? What do gay and lesbian people call the person with whom they're in a relationship?

If the relationship is a dating relationship, gay people typically use *boyfriend* and *girlfriend* the way heterosexual people do. If the relationship is more significant—committed, live-in, and so forth—gay people generally call their partner in life their *partner*, as in "I'd like to introduce you to my partner. . . ." Some people also use the word *spouse* when introducing a partner.

I can't say *partner* is a word I'm all that fond of, for two reasons. First, it's potentially confusing, because *partner* can also mean "business partner." Second, *partner* doesn't do justice to the relationship I have with my partner, who is really better described as my husband. But we're not legally married, so *husband* isn't really appropriate, and *husband* can also prove to be confusing when both partners are men. Once in a conversation with my grandmother I referred to my partner as my husband, and she asked, "So what are you, the wife?" I explained that we were both husbands, but she wasn't buying it.

Back in the old days when I was growing up, gay people called their partners their *lovers*. That word had its own problems, but at least it wasn't so clinical, and it suggested something more fun than simply a contractual relationship, which is what I picture when I think of the word *partner*—or the phrase *significant other*, for that matter.

? Do gay and lesbian couples have pet names or nicknames for each other?

Like straight couples, gay and lesbian couples may call each other by endearments or nicknames when they're in the privacy of their own homes. The nicknames and endearments range from the catchall "darling" and "honey" to "Bunny," "Wonkie," and "Beanie." I never said gay people weren't just as goofy as straight people.

? Why do gay people hold hands in public?

Some gay people who hold hands in public do so to make the point that gay people should be allowed to hold hands in public just as many heterosexual couples choose to do without thinking twice.

But, in general, gay people who hold hands in public do so because they enjoy having that kind of physical connection with a person they care about.

Because of public hostility toward gay and lesbian people, particularly those gay men and women who display any kind of affection in public for a same-gender partner, most gay people rarely hold hands in public without first considering where they are and whether holding hands would be a safe thing to do.

? What kinds of relationship problems do gay people have that result from being gay?

All couples, gay and straight, face challenges. Gay and lesbian people face some extra challenges, not the least of which is a world that is still fundamentally unwelcoming of same-gender couples. For example, gay and lesbian couples are less likely than heterosexual couples to have the support of their families, religious institutions, or the government (unless you live in a place where couple relationships between people of the same gender are legally sanctioned). Add to that society's expectation that gay relationships can't possibly last and the relative dearth of visible role models, and it begins to seem miraculous that there are any gay and lesbian couples at all.

? Why do gay people want to get married?

Not all gay and lesbian people think legal marriage is such a great idea, especially given how badly it seems to work out for so many heterosexual couples. But, in general, gay people think that legal marriage should be available to those gay and lesbian couples who wish to be legally married.

Those gay people who would like to legally marry would like to do so for all the same reasons that most couples choose to marry: first and foremost because they love each other, and along with that they want the legal and financial protections and benefits that will allow them to take care of one another and their children.

The legal protections and benefits of marriage are considerable. For example, in the case of death or medical emergency, the married spouse is the legal next of kin, which means he or she can make all decisions regarding medical care and funeral arrangements. And the next of kin are automatically granted hospital visitation rights.

In most states, married couples have the legal right to be on each other's insurance and pension plans. Married couples also get special tax exemptions and deductions and are eligible for

Social Security survivor's benefits. A married person may inherit property and may have automatic rights of survivorship that avoid inheritance tax. Married couples can routinely adopt a child jointly. And marriage laws offer legal protection in the event that a relationship comes to an end, providing for an orderly distribution of property.

For gay and lesbian couples who are raising children, the absence of state-sanctioned marriage can lead to all kinds of legal problems. (For more on this subject, see chapter 4, "Family and Children.")

And finally, there is the kind of dilemma faced by a couple like Charlene, who is a U.S. citizen, and Sandrina, who is French. Shortly after Sandrina arrived in the United States to get her master's degree in English literature, she met Charlene. Following a six-month courtship, they moved in together, hoping they could figure out a way for Sandrina to stay in the United States after she graduated.

For a heterosexual couple, marriage would have been a natural solution. If Charlene and Sandrina could marry, Sandrina would be eligible for citizenship and would be allowed to live and work in the United States. After exhausting all her legal options, Sandrina chose to remain in the United States with Charlene illegally. Both women live in fear that Sandrina will be discovered and deported.

? Can gay people get legally married? Where?

Yes, gay people can get legally married, but this issue is extremely fluid, so this is not the place to look for the latest information on which countries, and which states and provinces within those countries, have laws that permit gay people to marry. So I suggest you visit the Web site for the Human Rights Campaign (www.hrc.org), which contains extensive and up-to-date information—state-by-state and country-by-country—on the marriage rights issue.

In the United States, the first state to extend marriage rights to couples of the same gender was Massachusetts. The 2004 court decision that cleared the way for these marriages set off a furious political and social debate that will no doubt reverberate for years to come. In July 2000, Vermont became the first state in the United States to permit "civil unions" for couples of the same gender, which are legal marriages, except in name.

In Europe, the first country to extend marriage rights (not just equivalent or similar rights) to gay people was the Netherlands, in 2001.

? Are "civil unions" and "domestic partnerships" the same as legal marriage?

The only thing consistent about these two phrases is that they mean different things in different places, so you have to pay careful attention to what exactly you're committing to—and what, if any, legal rights you're gaining—if you're a gay couple and choose to make a legal commitment using a government-issued document.

For example, the city of New York allows nonmarried couples, both gay and straight, to register as "domestic partners." This largely symbolic gesture gives nonmarried couples who choose to register their relationships the opportunity to go on record as being a committed couple. Domestic partners are not granted the legal rights that are conferred on legally married couples (only states have the right to issue marriage licenses), although a domestic partner certificate may be necessary to qualify for family benefits for gay and lesbian spouses from employers, insurance companies, and even health clubs where such benefits are offered.

On what grounds do people oppose legal marriage for gay and lesbian couples?

People oppose extending legal marriage to gay men and lesbians because of their religious convictions, because of their political views, and because of ignorance and prejudice. Among the arguments I've heard most frequently in recent years are that marriage between people of the same gender is contrary to five thousand years of Western tradition, that it goes against the Bible and God's law (i.e., God created Adam and Eve, not Adam and Steve), and that it will devalue heterosexual marriage, destroy the American family, and lead to the legalization of polygamy and bestiality.

Everyone is entitled to his or her opinions, no matter how misguided I may think they are. But the facts don't bear out the claims made by those who would deny gay people the right to legal marriage. Whole books have been written on this subject, so I'll leave the extended debates to others. But I'd like to address a few of the more absurd claims.

I agree that marriage between two people of the same gender is generally not consistent with five thousand years of Western history, but then neither is marriage as we know it today. Marriage based on romantic love and free choice is a modern invention. Marriage customs have evolved dramatically over the millennia, and to suggests that such customs have remained static or have always reflected our contemporary ideas is not only misleading, it's a lie.

We should all be grateful that we aren't required to live by strict biblical law, including the laws that govern marriage. You don't believe me? Have a look at the Bible.

Regarding the devaluation of heterosexual marriage and the destruction of the American family, I have yet to hear a single coherent explanation from anyone regarding exactly *how* legal marriage between people of the same gender would accomplish this. I'm convinced that the reason no one is able to offer a rational or even vaguely intelligent response to that question is that there is none.

Interestingly, some of the very same religious and political leaders who in the past claimed that gay men, in particular, were promiscuous hedonists incapable of having lasting relationships are now among the most vocal opponents of extending marriage rights to gay people.

? Do gay people believe in polygamy and bestiality?

If there is one stupid question in this book, this is it. But it's here because some of the more extreme gay-marriage opponents (including elected officials of national stature) have suggested that granting gay people the right to legally marry will put us on a slippery slope that will inevitably lead to legalizing polygamy and bestiality. The last time I checked there was no organized effort among gay people to legalize polygamy and bestiality. But I do wonder about the interest of people who are obsessed with this issue.

? For gay and lesbian couples who live in places where they can't get married or places that don't offer civil unions or domestic partnerships, how can they protect each other, their children, and their property?

There are several legal documents that gay and lesbian couples can complete that give them some of the legal rights granted to heterosexual married couples. These include a will; a durable power of attorney, which allows you to designate a particular individual as the person you want to make medical and financial decisions for you should you become incapacitated; and joint-ownership agreements.

You can also draw up a legal letter, which my attorney calls a *designation of preference,* in which you state, for example, that you want your partner to be the first person to visit you should you be confined to an intensive-care unit. A hospital does not have to honor such a document, but the letter, along with the support of your doctor, may just do the trick.

? What do gay and lesbian couples do when they have to fill out medical or government forms that ask if they're married, single, or divorced?

At least when it comes to government forms, you answer honestly. If you've been with your partner for a decade but you're not legally married, it is best to check the box marked "single." With medical forms or other forms where I know I'm not risking getting stopped at the border, I always add a category for "partner" and check it off and write in my partner's name on the line marked "spouse."

The form that drives me up a wall is the U.S. immigration form, which asks how many family members you're traveling with. On trips out of the country, my partner and I almost always travel together, but because in the eyes of the law I'm traveling alone, I write in "zero." It's a small thing, but it's a pointed and galling reminder that my partner and I are second-class citizens.

? Can gay people get medical insurance at work for their partners?

It depends upon where you live and where you work, but an ever-increasing number of private companies, universities, and city and state governments offer the same benefits—including medical insurance—to the spouses of gay and lesbian employees that they offer to heterosexual married couples.

? What happens when one partner gets sick and goes to the hospital? Can the other partner visit and make medical decisions?

If you've got your papers in order (papers that should include a living will), yes, and this goes for all nonmarried couples, gay and straight. But if you don't, you could wind up living the nightmare that Sharon Kowalski and Karen Thompson faced after a 1983 car accident that left Kowalski brain damaged and quadriplegic. It took Thompson seven years to be named guardian, over the objections of Kowalski's parents, who were the legal next of kin. The Kowalskis also barred Thompson from visiting their daughter's nursing home for several years after the accident.

What took Karen Thompson seven years to achieve would likely have been granted quickly if the two women had drawn up a durable power of attorney (although the parents could have attempted to challenge this). And both guardianship and visitation rights would have been granted automatically if they'd been allowed to legally marry in the first place.

? What kinds of ceremonies do gay and lesbian couples have to celebrate their relationships? Why do they do it?

Because there is no gay-specific wedding tradition, gay couples celebrate their relationships in a range of ways, from exchanging rings in private to pull-out-all-the-stops events that may include a religious ceremony, matching tuxedos or dresses, traditional vows, a formal reception for two hundred, and a four-tiered wedding cake topped with two grooms or two brides.

Gay and lesbian couples have many different reasons for celebrating their relationships, but most mirror those of heterosexual couples, whether the celebration is an opportunity to formalize a commitment to each other in front of friends and family or a plain and simple declaration of mutual love.

? What's a gay wedding or commitment ceremony like?

No two ceremonies are exactly alike, so I'll tell you about the first gay commitment ceremony I attended back in 1992 for my friends Bill and Henry. The two men, who were both in their late twenties, had been together for nearly three years and had been formally engaged for a year (they bought each other identical watches for their engagement).

The invitation stated that Bill and Henry wanted me to join them for a ceremony celebrating their commitment to each other. The invitation went beyond the usual date, place, and time to explain what would happen at the ceremony. "We knew that most of the people we invited had never been to a gay commitment ceremony before," explained Henry. "We thought that the best way to make them comfortable was to spell out in the invitation what to expect. So in the invitation we said there would be an exchange of vows and rings, readings by several different people, and then a reception."

I don't know quite what I expected, but Bill and Henry's ceremony, which they held in their new apartment, was the most moving "wedding" I've ever been to—other than my own. (I've put *wedding* in quotes because Bill and Henry didn't call it a wedding, but in almost all ways, except for the fact the two men couldn't get a marriage license, that's what it was.)

Bill and Henry conducted the ceremony themselves. They were flanked by their parents. Both stated their love for each other and their mutual commitment before exchanging traditional gold wedding bands. Then Henry's mother and father spoke, as did Bill's father. By this time I was crying, as were most of the fifty people—friends, family, neighbors, both gay and straight—packed into Bill and Henry's living room. It was an incredibly emotional and loving ceremony, especially as various friends and family came up to speak. Then we all congratulated the dazed couple and feasted on Chinese food. The next day they left for their honeymoon.

I wasn't quite sold on the significance of a commitment ceremony before I attended Bill and Henry's. But it was clear to me from that event that the two men had entered a new stage of life—as do all married couples—by stating their vows and love for each other in the company of those people most important to them.

It wasn't just my imagination that things were different for Bill and Henry after their ceremony. "Our parents treat us differently," said Bill. "There's no question now in their minds that we're a couple, and they don't hesitate to offer their advice, as they would to any married child and his spouse. Sometimes that's good, and sometimes that's not so good." Henry added, "The two of us also take the relationship even more seriously than we did before. It gives us a new sense of commitment and security."

? How do gay couples split up? Do they get divorced?

Gay and lesbian couples end their relationships in mostly the same ways married heterosexual couples do. It's just as painful and often as ugly, but because most gay couples can't legally marry, they can't legally divorce.

For couples who have been through a divorce, it may sound appealing at first to be rid of the legal hassle of filing for divorce. Dream on. Without the legal protections that are built into marriage in the event of a divorce, dividing up property and arranging custody where children are involved can lead to legal and emotional nightmares even greater than the messiest heterosexual divorce.

? What should you do if you've fallen in love with a gay person but you're not gay?

If you're straight, it's not a great idea to fall in love with a gay person, because your feelings won't be reciprocated. If you can't help it and find yourself fantasizing about "turning" your gay or lesbian love interest straight, you should consider seeing a professional counselor to explore what drives you to pursue someone who is fundamentally unavailable.

Do gay people marry straight people? Why?

Many gay and lesbian people marry heterosexual people, and for a variety of reasons. Some do so because they believe it's the right thing to do based on what their parents, religion, and society have told them they should do. They want to "fit in" and live a "normal life," hoping to fulfill family or professional expectations.

Quite a few gay men and lesbians at the time they marry an opposite-gender spouse are in denial about their sexuality. Or they may simply not be fully aware of their feelings of same-gender attraction, a situation that seems to be true more often for women than for men. For example, when Katie married at the age of eighteen, she loved her husband, but she knew she "felt different from other girls," she explained.

Katie went on to tell me, "It wasn't until I'd been married for seven years and had four children that I had my first adult crush on a woman. And would you believe it was a woman in the church choir? Even after Mary and I became sexually involved, it still took me another year to admit to myself that I was a lesbian. I couldn't even say the word!"

Some gay people who marry partners of the opposite gender get married with the hope that they'll "get over" their feelings of same-gender sexual attraction. That was exactly what Edward hoped for when he married Suzanne. "We were both very young," said Edward, "and neither of us knew much of anything about homosexuality. I even told Suzanne that I had these feelings, but the psychiatrist I was seeing reassured us I would get over it, and that the best thing I could do was get married and have children."

Six years after they married, shortly after the birth of their second daughter, and after ten years of seeing the same psychiatrist, Edward ended the marriage. "I didn't get over it," he said. "In fact, by the time I left my wife—and fired my psychiatrist—I couldn't have been more certain that I was gay and that my psychiatrist was a quack."

Though some gay and lesbian people, like Edward, inform their opposite-gender spouses beforehand about their same-gender sexual orientation, most don't.

? How do heterosexual spouses react when they find out their wife or husband is gay?

According to Amity Pierce Buxton, author of *The Other Side of the Closet,* a book about the coming-out crisis for heterosexual spouses of gay and lesbian people, straight spouses greet the disclosure as a denial of the relationship.

"Shocked spouses," she writes, "typically feel rejected sexually and bereft of the mates that they thought they had. . . . Although relieved to know the reason behind changes in their partner's behavior or problems in marital sex, most feel hurt, angry and helpless."

And while their homosexual spouses most often feel relief stepping out of the closet, and are likely to receive support from other gay and lesbian people, the heterosexual spouses suddenly find themselves in a closet of their own, fearful of telling anyone the truth about their gay or lesbian spouse.

? Can the marriage survive?

Again, I defer to Amity Pierce Buxton, who explains, "Although a number of couples succeed in preserving the marriage, the majority do not. Despite sincere efforts, the sexual disparity, competition for the partner's attention or unconventional—and for some, immoral—arrangements eventually become intolerable for most spouses."

? What should you do if you think your spouse is lesbian or gay?

Before you do anything, find someone you can confide in, preferably a counselor who has experience dealing with your circumstance. Depending upon where you live, you may be able to find a support group for heterosexual people who have—or have had—homosexual spouses. (Visit the Web site for the Straight Spouse Network: www.ssnetwk.org.) You should also get your hands on a copy of *The Other Side of the Closet,* which is listed in the bibliography at the back of this book.

? What should you do if you're gay and your straight spouse doesn't know?

I often receive e-mail from people who find themselves in this circumstance but can't think of a way out. Frequently they'll speak of wanting to kill themselves because they can't imagine going on in a marriage where they have to pretend to be someone they're not but they also can't imagine hurting their spouses and breaking up their families.

My advice to people who find themselves in this circumstance is virtually always the same as in the previous question. You have to find help, because you can't get through this on your own. So, if you can, find a counselor who has experience dealing with gay people in an affirmative way and/or contact a local support group to find other people who have been through what you're going through.

? Do gay men and lesbians ever marry each other? Why?

Yes, there are gay men and lesbians who have married each other and even had children together in order to appear heterosexual. Some people do it because of their careers—men and women in the military, for example—others to gain citizenship, and others, still, because of family pressures.

I remember one of my college classmates who came from a very prominent and wealthy family. From what she knew about her parents, she assumed they would never let her take over the family business if they discovered she was a lesbian, so she set out to find and marry a gay man with a similar need to appear heterosexual.

I should also add that there are gay and lesbian people who are in denial about their sexual orientation, marry each other unknowingly (or knowingly, but subconsciously), and discover during the course of their marriage that both are homosexual.

7

Sex

? Do gay people have sex? If so, what do they do?

This reminds me of a favorite Marcus family story. One day, when my sister was about eight years old and on a weekend visit with our grandparents, she asked Grandma May whether grandmas had sex. My Jewish grandmother, who was quite Episcopalian in her manner and outlook, said, without skipping a beat or blushing, "Heidi, grandmas are just like everyone else." And that was the end of the conversation, whether my sister liked it or not.

Yes, like everyone else, gay people have sex, although I'm not sure everyone would agree on exactly what constitutes sex. Years ago, a young straight guy asked me what gay people consider "having sex." Before answering, I asked him what he considered having sex. He told me that for him having sex meant intercourse with a woman. Everything else was "just fooling around."

Like many people, I prefer a broader definition of what it means to have sex. In my mind, having sexual relations includes all the things we do to stimulate each other sexually. And no matter what your sexual orientation, this includes all the various things that make humans feel sexually aroused: looking at each other, talking, kissing, holding hands, massaging each other, licking each other, and so forth.

Of course, some things feel better than others, because some parts of the body are naturally more sensitive, like nipples, breasts, buttocks, lips, the clitoris, penis, and anus—and for some people, that tender spot on the back of the neck or behind the knees. And people use all kinds of things to stimulate the parts that feel good, including fingers, hands, tongue, mouth, penis, toes; you name it, people use it.

Having sex may or may not include reaching orgasm. And just as there are all kinds of ways to stimulate each other sexually, there are all kinds of ways to reach orgasm.

Needless to say, when you choose to have sex with another person, it's extremely important before you have sex to learn about sexually transmitted diseases, including HIV/AIDS, and to take the necessary precautions to prevent their spread—and heterosexuals need to know about birth control. (See the "Resources" section at the back of this book for information on how to learn more about HIV/AIDS and other sexually transmitted diseases.)

? Do gay people have sexual intercourse? How?

Yes, gay people can have sexual intercourse, but not penile-vaginal intercourse. Two men can, if they choose, have anal intercourse—insertion of the penis of one man into the anus of the other. Two women, if they desire vaginal penetration, can use fingers, a dildo, or whatever feels good to them.

Some lesbians who desire the experience of intercourse use a dildo attached to a waist harness that allows one woman to have intercourse with another woman. Some heterosexual women also use this method to engage in anal intercourse with their male partners.

Why do some gay men have anal intercourse and others don't?

It's all a matter of personal preference. Some gay men find anal intercourse a pleasurable sexual activity and others don't (just as some heterosexual people like and engage in anal intercourse and some don't—and for much the same reasons).

Gay men I've spoken with who don't engage in anal intercourse, either as the one doing the penetrating or the one being penetrated, offered a number of reasons for their preferences. Some men find it physically uncomfortable to be anally penetrated by a penis, or they don't enjoy assuming what has been traditionally viewed as a passive role. Other men choose not to engage in anal intercourse because of concerns about cleanliness, fears of contracting sexually transmitted diseases (even with the use of a condom), or moral concerns.

How can a lesbian be sexually satisfied (i.e., achieve orgasm) without a penis during sexual relations?

Any woman—gay or nongay—can tell you that a penis is not required to achieve an orgasm, and that penile-vaginal intercourse does not guarantee that a woman will have an orgasm.

What is usually required to achieve orgasm is stimulation of the clitoris, which is located outside and above the vagina, and/or of the G-spot, which is located inside the vagina.

The clitoris can be stimulated by using a number of different things, including fingers, the mouth, or a vibrator. And if a woman desires vaginal stimulation, a penis isn't required, because there are many different ways to penetrate and stimulate the vagina without a penis.

? Do gay people feel guilty about having sex with each other?

Some do and some don't. It depends upon an individual's experience, background, and beliefs. For example, by the time I became sexually active, I knew I preferred men, but I also knew that according to everything I had learned, homosexuality was wrong. So, of course I felt guilty about doing something wrong. But my guilt didn't override my innate desires, and over time the guilt faded.

Feelings of guilt don't fade for everyone. One man wrote to me for advice about his boyfriend, who was devoutly Catholic. He said, "Every time after we have sex, barely a second after he has an orgasm, he's out of bed, on his knees, genuflecting and begging God for forgiveness." The relationship didn't last.

Guilt is not everyone's experience. As Sonya, a middle-aged businesswoman from Atlanta, explained to me, the first time she was with a woman she didn't feel guilty at all. She said, "Making love to a woman felt like the most perfectly natural thing in the world for me. I was thirty-two. This was what I wanted. I'd waited all my life for it. Why in heaven's name would I feel guilty? I felt like going out and celebrating!"

Are lesbians virgins? How do gay men lose their virginity?

This question reminds me of a conversation I had with a woman friend in college. Long after she told me about all the fun she'd been having with her new boyfriend, she said she intended to remain a virgin until she married. I was more than a little perplexed. I thought back over our earlier conversations about how her boyfriend had done this to her or how she had done that to him. There was plenty of talk about what I thought sounded like passionate, sweaty, messy, lusty sex.

So I asked my friend how she could define herself as a virgin after all that sex. "I've never had intercourse," she explained. Of course! She was indeed technically a virgin, but only because she had never had a penis in her vagina. By her own description, her boyfriend's penis had been almost everywhere else.

Using the penile-penetration definition of virginity doesn't work quite so well for gay men and lesbians. (I don't think it works so well for heterosexuals either, but I'll leave that for others to debate.) For example, is a sexually active lesbian who has never had intercourse with a man still a virgin? Is she still a virgin if she has penetrated her partner's vagina with a dildo? Is a sexually active gay man who has never been penetrated anally by another man still a virgin? What if he has penetrated another man but has never been penetrated himself?

Given the realities and complexities of sexual relations between humans, I think it's time to get rid of the concept of virginity. And now let's move on to a really serious question!

Do gay men have bigger sexual appetites than straight guys?

Yes, we are sex machines. Oh, and our penises are bigger, too. Much bigger.

The truth, however, is dull to report. Gay men and heterosexual men are different only in whom they desire, not how much they desire. (Nor are they any different when it comes to the size of their penises.) Men, in general, have a range of sexual appetites, from never hungry to never satisfied.

Do gay men have more sexual partners than other people?

If you believe what some people say about gay men, you would think that all gay men have had a thousand or more sexual partners by the time they're thirty. Some very sexually active men—gay and straight—*have* had a thousand sexual partners by the time they're thirty.

My heterosexual male friends would argue—and have argued—that it's easier for gay men to have that many sexual partners than for straight men because men are more inclined than women to have sex with anything that moves. Maybe that's true, but from what I hear from single gay guys around the country, most feel lucky if they can get a date on Saturday night.

Are gay people more likely to get sexually transmitted diseases?

Sexually active people who don't make the effort to learn about sexually transmitted diseases and then protect themselves accordingly are at far greater risk of contracting a sexually transmitted disease, including HIV/AIDS, than someone who learns the facts and takes the recommended precautions. Viruses and germs don't care if you're gay or straight. They're just looking for a warm body.

? Didn't a lot of gay men die from AIDS? Is it a disease that only gay men get?

Let's start with what HIV/AIDS is. AIDS (acquired immunodeficiency syndrome) is a disease of the immune system that, if left untreated, eventually destroys the body's ability to fight other diseases. AIDS is caused by a virus, HIV (human immunodeficiency virus), which can be transmitted when blood, semen, or vaginal secretions containing the virus are passed from one person to another through, for example, unprotected (i.e., no condom) vaginal or anal intercourse or through intravenous drug use when needles are shared.

In the United States, HIV first entered the population in the late 1970s through gay men in New York City, Los Angeles, and San Francisco. And it spread very quickly, primarily within the gay male population, before the vast majority of gay and non-gay people knew what was happening and knew how to prevent the disease's spread. In the early years of the AIDS epidemic in the United States, the majority of people who became infected and died of the disease were men who had sex with other men.

Worldwide, the majority of people who have contracted HIV have been—and are—heterosexual. HIV/AIDS does not discriminate. It's an equal-opportunity disease that infects people who fail to use the well-understood methods to prevent its spread.

? Why are gay men still getting infected with HIV when we know how to prevent its spread?

Ah, this is the million-dollar question—but it really applies to all people, not just gay men. Most people become infected with HIV because they fail to do what's necessary to protect themselves. Why they fail to do so is the subject of much discussion and debate, and though this discussion could easily fill a book, I'll attempt to provide a brief overview here. First a story.

I had a conversation a while back with an acquaintance who is very well educated, in the heart of middle age, and a real enthusiast about life. He told me about how he had unprotected anal intercourse with a young man he had just met. My jaw was already on the floor before he got to the part where he told me, "And he ejaculated inside me." I was astonished—no, horrified. "How could you do that?" I asked. This man, who has read all the same articles I have and knows people who have died from AIDS, said, "It felt like the right thing to do. I trusted him. He told me that he'd tested negative [for HIV]." Right, and the check is in the mail.

In the heat of passion, people—gay and nongay, young and old—are not always entirely rational, especially when alcohol and/or drugs are part of the mixture. So sometimes even people who know better don't follow recommended guidelines for preventing the spread of HIV/AIDS. This is especially true of young people, who tend to feel immortal.

But besides thinking they'll live forever, many young gay men view AIDS as a disease that belongs to an older generation, and many heterosexuals mistakenly believe that AIDS is a disease that affects only gay men. Also, because younger people most often don't know anyone who has AIDS or has died from

AIDS and think they don't know anyone infected with HIV, they believe they're free from the risk of infection.

Other gay men don't take the appropriate precautions because they can't acknowledge to themselves that they're gay and engaging in sex with other men, even if that's what they're doing. (See the question in chapter 1 regarding "on the down low.") Because they don't think they're gay, and may mistakenly assume that AIDS is a "gay disease," they think they're not at risk.

This kind of thinking may sound far-fetched, but there are many men in very deep denial about who they are and what they're doing. This is an especially acute problem for African-American and Hispanic men, who are even more reluctant than white men to acknowledge that they're gay because of the more extreme condemnation of homosexuality in their communities. This is also an acute problem for their heterosexual wives or girlfriends, who may have no idea that they're in danger of being infected with HIV by their allegedly straight male partners who are engaging in sexually risky behavior with other men.

And finally, some people mistakenly assume that, with more effective treatments available for those infected with HIV, AIDS is no big deal and not worth the effort of taking proper precautions. But until there's an effective cure for AIDS, it's hard to imagine anyone realistically thinking that AIDS is no big deal.

Whatever the specific reason for not taking the appropriate precautions, gay men—like all other people, gay and straight—are only human, and humans do all kinds of things they know are dangerous, like smoking, driving without a seat belt, and drinking too much. Everyone likes to believe "it won't happen to me." But it can and it does.

? Where can you get more information on sexually transmitted diseases, including HIV/AIDS, and how to protect yourself?

See the "Resources" section at the back of this book.

? Do gay people use sex toys and look at pornography?

Ask any purveyor of sex toys about who buys and uses the various sexual implements available, and you'll find out that all kinds of people, male and female, gay and nongay, old and young, religious and agnostic, use sex toys—with each other and by themselves.

The same goes for pornography, but a quick scan of what's available will reveal that there's a much larger market for pornography that appeals to gay men and straight men than to lesbians or heterosexual women.

? If a lesbian uses a dildo, doesn't that imply she wants to be with a man?

No. A lesbian who uses a dildo is simply choosing to enjoy that type of vaginal or anal stimulation. It's really no different than when a straight man chooses to use a dildo to stimulate his anus. He's using the dildo because he enjoys how it feels, not because he wants to have intercourse with a man.

? What are "tops" and "bottoms"?

When a gay man refers to himself as a "top" or a "bottom," what he's saying is that he prefers to be the one doing the penetrating during anal intercourse—a "top"—or that he prefers to be penetrated—a "bottom." The distinction between tops and bottoms is also made among some lesbians, where a "top" uses a dildo or other implement to penetrate a "bottom."

Some people also use the "top" and "bottom" labels for the person who takes the aggressive versus the passive role when having sex of any kind.

Although some gay men and lesbians strictly define their sexual roles as "tops" or "bottoms," most do not use these labels and are likely to shift from more aggressive to less aggressive roles during sexual relations from minute to minute, day to day, week to week.

? Do gay couples have less sex over time?

Just like heterosexual people in couple relationships, most gay and lesbian people in couple relationships have less sex with each other over time.

? Can gay people have sex with someone of the opposite gender? Is it pleasurable?

Many gay and lesbian people have had sex with someone of the opposite gender. And though sex with someone of the opposite gender may not have been our first choice, for many gay and lesbian people there was certainly pleasure in the experience.

? Do gay people find members of the opposite sex physically unattractive?

The fact that you have feelings of sexual attraction for people of the same gender doesn't mean that you are physically repulsed by the opposite gender. Most gay and lesbian people simply don't have significant feelings of sexual attraction for members of the opposite sex.

When I first told some of my straight male friends at college that I was gay, a couple of them assumed I found women physically repulsive. I explained to them my thoughts on this by telling them a story about my girlfriend in summer camp when I was ten or eleven.

Eva had brown hair, green eyes, and a beautiful body. She was pretty, fun, and adventuresome. We had a great time together. We even held hands. But when the other boys talked about trying to get to first or second base with their girlfriends, I remember thinking that I'd rather play cards. If the other boys hadn't mentioned it, the possibility of getting sexual with Eva never would have occurred to me—but I certainly wasn't repulsed by her.

? What are gay bathhouses and sex clubs? Who goes to them and why?

Gay male bathhouses and sex clubs are two different things. A gay bathhouse is typically set up like a health club and may have a weight room, TV room, sauna, steam room, swimming pool, and other amenities. It may also have cubicles with beds that you can rent. When you enter a bathhouse you're assigned a locker for your clothes and given a towel.

The reason gay men go to bathhouses is generally to have sex, not lift weights. So once your clothes are in your locker, the search for a sexual partner or partners begins. As far as I know, there is no lesbian equivalent to gay male bathhouses.

Sex clubs are clubs where people go to have sex. The club may have a permanent location or a temporary location that changes from week to week. Some are by invitation only and others have strict entry requirements based on specific physical attributes. Some sex clubs are strictly for gay men, some for lesbians (although sex clubs are generally not nearly as popular among lesbians), some for both, and some for heterosexual people. In major cities, if you have a sexual desire, you can usually find a sex club where you can satisfy it, no matter what your sexual orientation.

? Why do gay men have sex in public bathrooms and parks? Do lesbians?

Historically, public parks and restrooms were just about the only places besides gay bars where men could find other men for sexual encounters. And though frequenting public parks and restrooms meant risking arrest by undercover police, such places allowed for even greater anonymity than did gay bars. In the days when almost all gay people kept their homosexuality a secret, anonymity was a key concern.

While gay men can now find sexual partners in lots of places, including online, some continue to seek out and engage in sex in public places. Men who do this give several reasons for engaging in public sex. Some men find this kind of sexual encounter convenient and quick. As one man explained, "There's no negotiating. You don't have to buy anyone a drink. You don't have to figure out whose home you're going to go to. You don't even have to say a single word."

Other men find the sense of danger inherent in public sex to be sexually exciting. Others like watching other men engage in sex. And still others want the anonymity of public sex because they're in a married heterosexual relationship, deeply closeted, or involved in a couple relationship with another man.

In general, lesbians do not engage in public sex. But all kinds of people—gay and nongay, men and women—at one time or another have had sex in public parks, restrooms, and airplanes, on beaches, and anywhere else you can imagine.

8

Work and the Military

? What kinds of jobs do gay people have?

Every kind of job that you can imagine, but because lots of gay people still fear for their jobs—because of prejudice and discrimination—many keep their sexual orientation a secret, or at least don't talk about their lives outside of work with their colleagues.

? Are there professions that attract large numbers of gay people?

Anecdotally, it would seem so. For example, it appears that a disproportionate number of male nurses, flight attendants, and dancers are gay. And it seems that a disproportionate number of female athletes, gym teachers, and military personal are lesbians. (There are no hard statistics, so I'm out on a limb here.)

I've heard a number of possible explanations for this apparent phenomenon. I don't think any one explanation is adequate, but in the absence of any concrete answers, some of the explanations I've come across are worth considering.

One theory I've heard is that gay men enter traditionally female professions and lesbians enter traditionally male professions in larger numbers than their heterosexual counterparts because gay men and lesbians are more likely to feel comfortable about crossing gender lines to do the kind work they prefer. Another theory is that gay and lesbian people are attracted to fields that have typically overlooked or been accepting of homosexuality, like the arts and the service professions.

One common stereotype is that gay men are attracted to certain jobs because gay men are more likely than straight men to be artistically gifted, and that lesbians are attracted to certain jobs because they're more likely than heterosexual women to be mechanically gifted. Sounds like a research opportunity here for an ambitious graduate student.

Of the many explanations I've heard, I think it's easiest to understand how the fear of discovery—or the negative experience of working in a profession where you have to hide your sexual orientation and live with the fear of discovery—has led gay people to pursue certain jobs or professions and to avoid others. The journalist and writer Frank Browning, who is something of an expert on matters concerning gay people, noted: "In the past, once you realized that you'd been sentenced to a homosexual life, you assumed that a lot of worlds were closed to you because of social expectations.

"There are forms of social performance that you're expected to meet, such as having a spouse and bringing a spouse to social functions. For this reason, many gay and lesbian people retreated into their own professional worlds and became florists or dog groomers or whatever. They pursued jobs and careers they could control, where they wouldn't be subject to someone else's judgment." Browning acknowledges that this is only a partial answer to a question that still remains to be adequately addressed.

? What are the popular stereotypes of the kinds of jobs gay people have?

Here are some of the stereotypes: Gay men are hairdressers, florists, nurses, elementary-school teachers, decorators, dancers, and childcare workers. Lesbians are gym teachers, professional athletes, truck drivers, construction workers, dog groomers, and members of the military.

It would be interesting to know if a disproportionate number of gay people do indeed fill the jobs that are thought of as stereotypically gay or lesbian, but no one really knows. And if it's found that gay and lesbian people do fill a larger percentage of these jobs than you would expect to find based on their numbers in the population, we're still left with the "why." Do gay men actually make better florists? Do lesbians make better gym teachers? I wonder.

I hasten to add that because gay and lesbian people work in every profession, you can't assume that all men who work in what we think of as typically macho jobs, like construction, are straight. Similarly, not all women who work in what we consider typically female jobs, like child care, are heterosexual. And, of course, there are plenty of heterosexual male flight attendants, dancers, and florists, and plenty of straight female gym teachers and athletes.

Are gay people more likely to pursue artistic careers?

It appears that gay men, at least, are more likely to pursue artistic careers than are heterosexual men. The AIDS crisis, which hit hardest among gay men in the United States during the 1980s through the mid-1990s, made this tragically clear, with a disproportionately high number of deaths from AIDS among the ranks of male dancers, actors, musicians, designers, and other artistic professionals.

But though gay men may be more prevalent in artistic professions in comparison to all other professions, there are plenty of heterosexual people who work in creative professions, including both the visual and performing arts.

Do gay people make more money than heterosexual people?

As a rule, no. Gay people, on average, are as diverse in the amount of money they earn as straight people. However, those gay and lesbian people who don't have children to support, like those heterosexual people who don't have children to support, have higher disposable incomes.

When it comes to gay and lesbian couples, there is a notable difference in combined income in comparison to heterosexual couples, whether or not there are children to support. Gay male couples are likely to have higher combined incomes than male-female couples, because two men are likely to earn more money than a man and a woman; on average, women are paid less than men.

By contrast, lesbian couples, on average, have lower combined incomes than male-female couples, because two women are likely to earn less money than a male-female household.

? Some people think gay men and lesbians should not be allowed to be teachers. What's their argument?

Stupidity and prejudice are behind their arguments, because there is no rational reason why gay people shouldn't be teachers. And the fact is that gay and lesbian teachers are already teaching in classrooms all across the country, as they have been for generations.

Those who object to gay teachers in the classroom base their arguments on the mistaken twin assumptions that lesbian and gay teachers are more likely to molest their students than heterosexual teachers and that gay teachers will set the wrong example and influence their students to become homosexuals.

First, regarding child molesting, see the answer to my question on this subject in chapter 1. I'd rather you read the whole answer than an abbreviated version here. Second, no one—not a teacher, a parent, or a favorite aunt—can influence anyone to "become" a homosexual, because sexual orientation is innate and immutable. (And if you don't know that by this point in the book, you haven't been paying attention.)

The best a gay or lesbian teacher can do is be an inspiring educator and set an example as a positive role model to all children—to show them that someone can be a gay or lesbian person and a good teacher. Plenty of us, including this writer, would have welcomed positive gay and lesbian role models as we struggled through school in isolation. Unfortunately for the teachers who taught when I was a young person, a teacher who was gay had to carefully guard his or her secret or risk almost certain dismissal.

I like what a lesbian comedian once said about this subject: "If teachers had that kind of influence over students, we'd all be nuns." The distinction here, of course, is that you may be able to persuade children to become nuns or priests. You cannot, however, convince anyone to become gay or lesbian.

? What about openly gay teachers?

Well, this is an interesting distinction, because even some people who support the idea of gay and lesbian teachers being allowed to teach aren't so keen on the idea of *openly* gay teachers being allowed to teach. In other words, they think it's okay as long as gay teachers leave the truth about their lives at the school's front door.

This is easier said than done. Think for a second what it would mean for any teacher to leave his or her sexual orientation at the door. For a heterosexual teacher that would mean not wearing a wedding band to class, because the wedding band is a generally recognized symbol of a heterosexual marriage (although as gay couples increasingly choose to wear wedding rings, you can't always assume that the person wearing the gold band has an opposite-gender partner).

Leaving the truth about your sexual orientation at the door would also mean that a teacher—gay or straight—could not bring a spouse to school social events or answer personal questions. Teachers are human, so inevitably their personal lives come up in class, particularly when students reach an age when they start asking teachers personal questions, like "Are you married?" or "Do you have a boyfriend?" A married teacher would have to say, "I can't talk about my personal life," which seems pretty silly when you think about it.

This issue goes beyond personal questions, as Ms. Shapiro, who teaches at a large high school outside Denver, explained to me. "What am I supposed to do when students call each other 'fag' and 'dyke'? Am I supposed to sit there and let them use words like that? Should I challenge them and tell them that saying 'fag' and 'dyke' is just as bad as saying 'nigger'? But then, because I'm defending gay people, my students might figure out I'm a lesbian. And if they figure out I'm a lesbian and someone complains to the administration, I could lose my job. Put yourself in my shoes. Would you like to live like that?"

? Are some places of employment more welcoming to gay people than others?

Yes. Increasingly, major corporations and smaller companies, as well as colleges and universities and other nonprofit institutions, are making an effort to welcome gay and lesbian people. They do this, for example, by prohibiting discrimination on the basis of sexual orientation, offering domestic-partner benefits, organizing diversity-training workshops (to familiarize employees with issues concerning race, gender, and sexual orientation), and supporting in-house gay and lesbian employee organizations.

In addition, a growing number of states and municipalities are providing domestic-partner benefits to gay employees. And, of course, gay and lesbian social-service agencies and organizations, as well as businesses owned and run by gay men and lesbians, welcome gay and lesbian employees.

Thc Human Rights Campaign (HRC) publishes an annual list of the best companies for gay and lesbian employees. I also suggest having a look at the HRC Web site (www.hrc.org) and the Lambda Legal Web site (www.lambdalegal.org) for information on domestic-partnership benefits.

❓ What happens when gay people come out at work or are found out?

Gay people who come out of the closet at work or are found out have a range of experiences, from complete acceptance to being fired. And for those gay people who are fired for being gay in places where gay people are not protected by law from discrimination, there is generally no recourse other than looking for another job.

A growing number of young gay people who have no interest in hiding their sexual orientation or pretending they're something they're not may choose to make clear in the job-interview process that they're gay. They do this either by including on their résumés their involvement with gay organizations or by bringing up the issue in interviews.

For example, when Ralph, a recent law school graduate, was interviewing for jobs, he decided to be up-front about his sexuality. So before he was made an offer at the firm where he had worked the previous summer, Ralph had a talk with the hiring partner.

As Ralph explained to me, "If there was going to be a problem, I wanted to know in advance so I could look for a job elsewhere. So I walked into the hiring partner's office and asked him if I could close the door. I told him that I sensed there was a good chance they would offer me a job, and that they should know something about my personal life before they hired me—that I was gay. He asked me why I thought it was important to tell him that, and I told him that I didn't want it to come out later and then be a problem. He looked at me and said that that was exactly *his* problem. He was gay and had always kept it a secret." Ralph was offered the job, and he accepted it.

Carolyn Mobley's experience was quite different. Now an associate pastor for a predominantly gay church in Houston, Carolyn was fired from an earlier job as a Christian educator because she was gay. When Carolyn first interviewed for that job, which was for an organization located in the heart of a low-income-housing community in Atlanta, no one asked her about her sexuality. But three years after she was hired, she was called into her boss's office and told that a student who had stayed in her home had come across some things that indicated she was a lesbian.

As Carolyn explained to me, "Their biggest accusation was that I wrote checks to a gay church and that this girl saw pictures of me in my photo album sitting on the hood of my car with my roommate, with my arms draped around her. My boss asked if I was a lesbian, and I said that he didn't have the right to ask me that. Then he said, 'If you can't tell us that you're not, we need your resignation.' I said, 'When do you want it?' It was clear to me there was no changing his mind."

Not everyone is either accepted or fired. Billie, a schoolteacher in a city near San Francisco, knows she won't be fired if her principal finds out she's a lesbian, in part because the city where she works forbids discrimination based on sexual orientation. "But I know they'll make my life so miserable that I'll have to quit," she said. "I hate living like this, but my partner is unemployed and I can't afford to lose my job. So there's no way I would come out, and I'm doing everything I can to make sure no one finds out."

Do some gay people have to hide their sexual orientation at work?

Yes. For instance, any gay man or woman who serves in the U.S. military has to hide his or her sexual orientation or risk almost certain dismissal. There are also plenty of other people, like Carolyn and Billie, whose situations I talked about in the previous question, who could risk their jobs or count on being harassed by coworkers if they revealed their sexual orientation, particularly if they work for a company or boss who is known to be hostile toward gay people. And there are still others who fear that their careers could be hampered by public disclosure of their sexual orientation, including politicians, corporate executives, professional athletes, and high-profile actors, actresses, and entertainers.

Are there places where gay people are protected by law from being fired solely because of their sexual orientation?

Fortunately, yes. Federal employees—other than those serving in the U.S. military—are protected from discrimination, as are people who live in the states and municipalities that have passed laws protecting gay people from discrimination based on sexual orientation. Also, a growing number of smaller companies, the vast majority of the Fortune 500 companies, and many colleges, universities, and other nonprofit organizations have incorporated sexual orientation into their nondiscrimination policies.

? What about gay people in the military?

There are two simple reasons gay people are routinely thrown out of the U.S. military for being gay: stupidity and prejudice—not on the part of the gay servicemen and women, but on the part of the people who run the military.

The U.S. military's current policy regarding gay people, which dates back to 1993, is known as "Don't Ask, Don't Tell." Loosely, this means: if you're gay, keep it a secret, and we won't bother you. Still, in the first ten years after the policy was put in place, more than ten thousand service members were thrown out of the military for failing to keep their secret a secret (this according to the Servicemembers Legal Defense Network [www.sldn.org], a gay rights group that monitors the armed services and provides assistance to service members hurt by the military's antigay policies).

As reported in the *New York Times,* among those discharged by the Pentagon between 1998 and 2003 for being gay were twenty service members who spoke or studied Arabic, "despite a critical shortage of translators and interpreters needed for the fight against terrorism." Makes you wonder about the Pentagon's priorities.

? Why does the U.S. military have a problem with gay people?

Senior officials in the U.S. military and political leaders have, over the years, come up with a long list of reasons why they first opposed lifting the long-standing ban on gay people in the military and, after 1993, why they opposed allowing gay people to serve openly.

The list of reasons includes the following: gay and lesbian people are security risks because they can be easily blackmailed by someone threatening to reveal their secret (a problem that would easily be solved by allowing gay people to serve openly); the presence of homosexuals in the force would be detrimental to good order and discipline, principally around the issue of privacy; the presence of gay people would seriously impair the accomplishment of military missions by undermining discipline, morale, and cohesiveness among the troops; if homosexuals were allowed to openly declare their sexual orientation, heterosexuals who shower with gay men would have an uncomfortable feeling of someone watching. (If servicemen are so fainthearted about the possibility of being looked at in the shower, the Pentagon should worry about how its soldiers will hold up on the battlefield.)

The problem with this long list of reasons given for discriminating against gay servicepeople is that the Pentagon's own studies have discredited these claims, as have the experiences of the nation's major allies, including Canada, Israel, and the members states of the European Union, where there is no discrimination against gay people serving in the military. In fact, the British Navy actively recruits gay people by advertising in gay and lesbian publications.

So when you set aside all the excuses offered up by the U.S. military and government officials for continuing to hold fast to its "Don't Ask, Don't Tell" policy toward gay service members, the only explanations left for this costly and wasteful policy are prejudice and stupidity. Plain and simple.

? Why do gay people join the military in the first place?

Gay and lesbian people join today's all-volunteer army for the same reasons that straight people do: pay, training, educational benefits, camaraderie, overseas travel, leadership challenges, and often a desire to serve their country. Some gay people in the military also say they want to prove that they can serve their country just as effectively as anyone else.

? Do gay people make good soldiers?

Several reports, including a number commissioned by the Pentagon itself, concluded that there was no evidence that homosexuals were any greater security risk than heterosexuals and that they were no more likely to be subject to blackmail. The reports also found no evidence that homosexuals disrupted the armed forces; in fact, they praised the performance of gay men and lesbians in the military and urged their retention.

? If you're fired from your job or thrown out of the military because you're gay, what can you do about it?

You can contact a local or national legal organization that specializes in gay rights cases, for example, Lambda Legal (www.lambdalegal.org). Or if you're in the military, contact the Servicemembers Legal Defense Network (www.sldn.org). See the "Resources" section at the back of this book for complete contact information.

? Are there gay people who keep their sexual orientation secret at work even though they don't have to?

There are lots of people who choose to keep their sexual orientation secret at work even when there is little, if any, real risk that their careers would be jeopardized if it were known that they are gay. And this includes people who work for companies or live in places that strictly forbid discrimination based on sexual orientation. These gay men and women choose to remain closeted for a couple of primary reasons.

First, some are simply accustomed to keeping their personal lives completely separate from their work lives. This includes many people who came of age at a time when being openly gay on your job was unthinkable. Second, some people choose to remain secretive because they fear the unknown. Will their colleagues be uncomfortable? What will their boss think? Will disclosure affect a promotion? These concerns can be especially acute when there are few—if any—colleagues who are openly gay. Not many people are willing to step into uncharted territory, especially if that means the possibility of jeopardizing their livelihood.

? Why do gay people want to be open about their sexual orientation at work?

In general, gay people would like to go about their lives in the same ways that heterosexual people do, and that includes not having to hide the facts of their relationships and personal lives from their colleagues. That may even include the wish to have a photo of their partner on their desk. For more on the subject of why gay people want to be open about their sexual orientation, see chapter 3, "Coming Out / Going Public."

Do they bring a same-gender date or spouse to company parties?

Lots of gay and lesbian people would like to bring a same-gender date or partner to their company's social events, and some do. But even for people who work at companies where gay people are welcome, not everyone feels comfortable bringing a same-gender partner to a social event, especially if they think they'll be the only gay couple.

My favorite story on this subject comes from my friends Daryl and Carlton, who were among the first people I knew who accompanied each other to school social events and, later, to work social events as a couple (they've been together since the late 1970s). This was in the years before there was a generally accepted word for what gay people called their partners. Carlton told me, "When Daryl took me to his architecture school graduation dinner party, he introduced me as his 'comrade' to all his professors. Everyone thought we were communists or something. It was embarrassing. By the end of the night I'd convinced him to use the word *spouse.*"

Can you be openly gay and succeed professionally?

Yes. And there are more and more examples with each passing year of openly gay and lesbian people reaching the top of their professions. There are, however, exceptions, most visibly the military and professional sports. (See chapter 14 for more information on gay people and sports). And, while an increasing number of politicians, corporate executives, movie and television actors, and other entertainers have come out about their sexual orientation, most who are at the highest levels of their professions remain hidden.

9

Where Gay and Lesbian People Live

? Where do gay and lesbian people live?

Everywhere, from rural North Carolina and southern Idaho to Juneau, Alaska. (And I know for a fact that there are gay people in these three places in particular, because I've interviewed gay couples.) However, large numbers of gay and lesbian people migrate from rural areas and small towns to cities and major metropolitan areas, so you're more likely to find larger concentrations of gay people, as well as find more organizations and resources for gay men and women, in New York City, Chicago, San Francisco, Houston, Atlanta, and Los Angeles than in Cicero, Indiana (where I know there is at least one gay person).

There's a very interesting book called *The Gay and Lesbian Atlas*, published in 2004 by Urban Institute Press, that offers a detailed look at the six hundred thousand same-sex couples who identified themselves in the 2000 U.S. census. The book's extensive analyses show that these couples live in 99.3 percent of U.S. counties and that, not surprisingly, large urban areas have high concentrations of same-sex couples, "but so do smaller metropolitan areas like Santa Fe, New Mexico; Portland, Maine; and Burlington, Vermont."

In addition, the book's authors, Gary J. Gates and Jason Ost, found that in a ranking of 1,360 American communities with more than fifty same-sex couples, the top three towns with the highest concentration of gay and lesbian couples are "more bucolic than bustling, more Mayberry than Manhattan." The top three, in descending order, are Provincetown, Massachusetts; Guerneville, California; and Wilton Manors, Florida. The next seven are West Hollywood, California; Palm Springs, California; Miami Shores, Florida; Decatur, Georgia; Key West, Florida; Northampton, Massachusetts; and North Druid Hills, Georgia.

? Why do so many gay people live in big cities?

Large cities in the United States have long been magnets for gay and lesbian people in search of other people like themselves, and for decades these cities have had significant gay and lesbian subcultures, including gay bars and clubs. These cities have in more recent years developed well-organized gay communities, complete with community centers, softball teams, choruses, and countless other social, religious, and professional organizations.

Big cities have also provided the kind of anonymity—and distance from home—that has allowed gay and lesbian people to keep their homosexual identities safely hidden, especially from their families. As gay people have grown more comfortable, and people everywhere have grown more accepting, increasing numbers of gay people are choosing to remain in or near the communities where they grew up, whether those communities are in major metropolitan areas or in smaller cities and towns.

Blighted city neighborhoods have also proven a draw for gay male couples in particular, who have been attracted by depressed housing prices and historic housing stock in need of renovation. These couples have been at the cutting edge of revitalization efforts in urban neighborhoods across the country as they've restored houses and opened new businesses.

? How did San Francisco become such a popular place for gay people to live?

One possible explanation for San Francisco's popularity among gay and lesbian people early on, besides its status as a major port city and its long-standing reputation for tolerating people who lead comparatively unconventional lives, was suggested to me by Judge Herbert Donaldson, whom I interviewed for my book *Making Gay History.*

As a young attorney, Donaldson was involved with an early gay rights organization in San Francisco called the Society for Individual Rights (SIR). SIR, along with other gay and lesbian organizations in San Francisco, planned a fund-raising ball for the evening of January 1, 1965. The ball turned into a major confrontation between the police, who didn't want the event to take place, and the hundreds of gay and lesbian people who were attending it. Several people were arrested, including Donaldson.

As Donaldson recalled, "The police made this estimate that there were seventy thousand homosexuals in the city. There weren't, but when they carry it on the [news] wire services that there are seventy thousand, you've got seventy thousand others out in the country who want to come and join that seventy thousand here! They're still coming."

By the 1970s, San Francisco's large and politically active gay and lesbian population, in combination with the city's reputation as a relatively friendly place for gay men and lesbians and its mild climate and physical beauty, made it a popular destination for gay people in search of a better life.

? Why do gay and lesbian people create their own neighborhoods?

Living in a community where there are lots of other gay people or where gay people make up the majority of residents is for some gay men and women preferable to living in places where they are the only—or among a relative handful of—gay individuals or couples.

Gay men and lesbians choose to live in these communities for many of the same reasons that people from different ethnic, racial, and religious groups choose to live in neighborhoods populated primarily by people like themselves: for comfort, a sense of community, safety, convenience, and because of discrimination. And for single men and women, a gay and lesbian neighborhood also offers more opportunities to meet and socialize with other gay people.

In San Francisco's Castro neighborhood, for example, many of the shopkeepers, as well as the doctors, dentists, and accountants, are gay or lesbian or they're gay-friendly, so you can be yourself and not worry about being judged. And if you want to buy a book like the one you're holding in your hands, there's a bookstore that specializes in books of interest to gay people. And if you want to buy a greeting card for a gay or lesbian couple you know who are celebrating an anniversary, there are plenty of places where you can find the appropriate greeting card.

In a neighborhood like the Castro, you also don't have to worry about discrimination. For example, if you're looking for an apartment with your same-gender partner, you aren't likely to encounter a landlord who doesn't rent to gay people.

? What are some gay neighborhoods, and what are they like?

Most major cities have neighborhoods that are popular with gay and lesbian people. For example, in Washington, D.C., it's the Dupont Circle neighborhood, which is also popular with young straight families and single people. In Los Angeles, it's West Hollywood, which is actually an incorporated city. In Chicago, it's Boystown. In New York City, it's Chelsea. In Houston, it's the Melrose neighborhood. And in Atlanta, lots of gay people have chosen to live in the Midtown neighborhood.

Most city neighborhoods popular with gay people look very much like any other neighborhood except that there are stores, restaurants, and bars that cater to and/or welcome a gay and lesbian clientele. You're also likely to see more identifiably gay and lesbian people on the street. And occasionally you'll see same-gender couples holding hands.

My partner and I live in a place that most people would identify as a gay neighborhood, and we really like living there. It's not that we even make up the majority of the residents, because we don't. (I'm guessing that we're about 30 or 40 percent of the total.) What we like is that in our neighborhood we're nothing special. When we go into a restaurant we're not the only gay people. Our neighborhood shopkeepers know that when I refer to my partner I'm not talking about my business partner. And all the service people we deal with, from the dry cleaner to the plumber, never look at us like we're aliens—and because of where we live I simply assume that that will always be the case. And what could be bad about that?

? What's it like for lesbians and gay men who live in places where there aren't a lot of gay people—in the suburbs or small towns, for example?

It really depends on the specific place you're talking about, because gay men and lesbians have had a range of experiences in the communities where they live, from very positive to very negative. It's tough to generalize.

Here's one example of a couple who had a mixed, although ultimately positive, experience: Connie and Renata decided to move from New York City to a suburban, almost rural, middle-class/working-class community. The two women, who had been together for nearly twenty years, didn't anticipate problems with their new neighbors, but because they were pretty certain they were the only gay couple to move into the area, they were a little apprehensive. "We thought we might have some problems," said Connie, "but we had our hopes up."

One afternoon a few months after they moved in, Connie and Renata found the word *dyke* spray-painted on their front door. "That scared us to death," said Renata, "but we decided to repaint the door and hope that it wouldn't happen again." It didn't—in part, they think, because they made a concerted effort to get to know their neighbors. "We hoped that once people got to know us, they'd treat us just like any other neighbors," said Connie.

Do they have any regrets? "No," said Renata. "This was something we wanted to do. We weren't twenty-five anymore, so we didn't care about nightlife. We just wanted peace and quiet and a backyard. That sounds hopelessly dull, but it's what we wanted. Maybe we should have done a better job of anticipating that not everyone would welcome us, but we've learned—and our neighbors have learned—from the experience."

Since I first interviewed Connie and Renata, two other gay couples have moved into the community, one with kids, so they're not nearly the curiosity they once were.

10

Socializing and Friends

? What do gay people talk about when they get together with gay friends?

In addition to talking about all the things that heterosexual people talk about, many gay and lesbian people talk about being gay and about the latest news on gay and lesbian rights issues—although how much gay people discuss these issues depends upon their stage in life. If you're in the process of getting coupled or you're working on having children, you're likely to discuss gay issues, legal issues in particular, far more than the average single gay person.

An acquaintance once asked me why gay people make such a big deal about being gay and talk about it all the time. I explained that once being gay is no longer a big deal within our society, and once our civil rights are no longer questioned, we'll likely stop talking about it.

? Do lesbians and gay men get along?

Some do. Some don't. But in general, whether gay men and gay women get along has more to do with individual personalities than anything else. There are plenty of long-lasting friendships between gay men and lesbians to disprove the stereotype that gay men and lesbians have an innate dislike for one another.

Historically, however, within the gay rights movement there were often tensions, and sometimes deep divisions, between lesbians and gay men. And often for good reasons. In the early days of the movement, back in the 1950s, many—if not most—gay men treated gay women the way most heterosexual men treated women. "They thought we were there to serve coffee and doughnuts," said one activist, now in her seventies.

Are there still gay men who as a rule profess a dislike for lesbians? And are there still lesbians who as a rule profess a dislike for gay men? Sure. Like everyone else, gay people are fully capable of prejudice.

? Do gay people have heterosexual friends?

Most do, but not all straight people who have gay friends are aware that their friends are gay. That's because not all gay people are comfortable revealing the truth about their sexual orientation. That can make friendship a little challenging, because keeping your sexual orientation secret requires leaving out information or making things up, neither of which is particularly good for building a strong friendship.

A small percentage of gay people choose not to have heterosexual friends. They may feel uncomfortable around straight people or may simply prefer only the companionship of other gay men and lesbians.

? Why do some heterosexual women have a lot of gay male friends?

This is a subject that seems to generate a lot of interest, and a consequently significant number of newspaper and magazine articles, books, films (including *The Object of My Affection* and *My Best Friend's Wedding*), and a hit television show, *Will and Grace*, which went on the air in the fall of 1998 and quickly became one of the most popular situation comedies in the United States.

I'll leave the psychological analysis to the mental health professionals, but I think my friend Sally offers some interesting—albeit a little harsh—insight based on her own experience. She said, "Many straight men are pigs. Seriously, I don't want to say anything that knocks straight men, but do you think I'll ever meet a straight man who likes the arts and gardening? Those are the things I talk to my gay friends about.

"Also, I find that my gay men friends have done a lot of soul-searching and self-examination, and that's made them empathetic people. And I know I can talk to them about life issues that involve not following the crowd. They're supportive of me and the risks I've taken with my life and work. And in general they're more understanding than my women friends. Women care about men. My gay friends care about me."

? If you think a friend is gay, but he or she hasn't said anything about it, what should you say?

If you're perfectly happy with your friendship, you don't have to say anything. But if you feel there's a barrier between you and your friend and you think the likely reason is your friend's hidden sexual orientation, you may want to bring it up by speaking with your friend or, if that seems too direct, writing a letter. (Because e-mail can easily be forwarded, by accident or on purpose, to half the world, I suggest a handwritten note. When it comes to discussions regarding sexuality, it never hurts to err on the side of discretion.)

If you're comfortable talking directly, you can ask your friend, "Are you gay?" Or you can say (or write), "You're my friend, and I care about you. I have the feeling there's something standing in the way of us becoming better friends. If it has anything to do with you being gay [or lesbian], I want you to know that if that's the case I'm perfectly comfortable and completely supportive."

Not everyone likes to take the direct approach, and not all gay people who are circumspect about their sexual orientation respond well to being confronted so directly. So you may choose to let your friend know that you're familiar with and supportive of gay people by mentioning something you saw on television that was sympathetic to gay people or something you read in the news about gay rights or prejudice that upset you. (And be prepared to talk about it in a knowledgeable way.) This gives your friend an opening if he or she chooses to be more forthcoming about his or her life.

Keep in mind that many gay and lesbian people assume that if their straight friends don't raise the subject, those friends either don't know or don't want to hear about their gay friend's life beyond what they already know. But if the letters and e-mails I've received over the years from heterosexual people concerned about their gay friends (who think their straight friends don't know they're gay) are any indication, there are a lot of straight people out there waiting for their gay friends to say something.

In general, these people have told me they've been reluctant to broach the subject with their gay friends because they assume their gay friends would bring it up if it were something they wanted to talk about. They don't want to be pushy or risk embarrassing their friends, so they don't say anything.

Of course, I also hear from gay people who are afraid of how their straight friends might react to the news that their friend is gay, and consequently they're reluctant to bring up the subject themselves. So the net result is that no one says anything and everyone winds up feeling uncomfortable, and the opportunity to have deeper friendships is delayed or lost entirely.

My suggestion is this: if you want to tell your gay friends—or friends you suspect are gay—that sexual orientation is not an issue for you, don't wait for your gay friends to bring it up. And the same goes for gay people: Don't wait for your straight friends to bring it up. There may be more to gain from the experience of being open than you might imagine.

? Why do gay people belong to social organizations and go to bars and clubs that are just for gay people?

Have you ever been in a room where you were the only one? The only woman, the only man, the only Jew, the only Muslim, the only black person, the only Asian person, or the only kid in a room full of adults? Well, then you know what if feels like to be different. And sometimes it's nice to be with people who are just like you, especially if the way in which you're different makes other people feel less than kindly toward you.

When you step into a gay or lesbian bar or play on an all-gay softball team, you're not an outsider. You can be yourself, which includes being physically affectionate in public in ways that heterosexual people take for granted (and get upset about when they see gay people doing the same things). There's no fear of being judged or discriminated against for being gay. At its best, the experience offers the sense of being with "family," in the most positive sense of the word.

For example, I remember when I attended the first conference of the newly founded National Lesbian & Gay Journalists Association back in the early 1990s. The experience was extraordinary. More than three hundred gay and lesbian journalists attended, and though there was plenty of disagreement about all kinds of professional and political issues, it was great to share experiences and ideas with gay journalists from across the country and the professional spectrum. For many who attended, the conference was their first opportunity to talk with other gay and lesbian journalists.

? What's a gay bar like?

First, it's important to understand that gay and lesbian bars have historically played a key role in gay social life, because for a long time bars were the only public places where gay people could meet and socialize. Though that's often no longer the case in most cities, bars still play an important role as gathering places for gay men and women.

There are all kinds of gay and lesbian bars, and they range from very attractive, well-designed, multistory confections to corner dives and everything in between.

In the nation's major cities, different bars cater to different kinds of people and different tastes. There are bars for men, women, older men, younger men; there are country-and-western dance bars, young professional bars, hustler bars, bars with back rooms (for those interested in sexual encounters), and leather bars (for people who like to dress up in black leather and have an interest in S&M—sadomasochistic sexual activities).

In smaller cities and towns there may be only one bar for everyone. On a visit to Juneau, Alaska, back in the late 1980s, I went to what was then that city's one gay and lesbian bar. It was at the back of a restaurant a few blocks from downtown. The bar itself was about six feet in length. There were eight stools and enough room for another eight people to stand. You had to meet everyone in the bar because there was no way not to. The bartender joked that the bar was gay only until someone heterosexual walked in.

? What kinds of social organizations do gay people have?

What kinds of social organizations *don't* gay people have? Check out the listings online or in local gay and lesbian publications around the country and you can find just about any gay social organization you can imagine, from gay and lesbian college fraternities and alumnae and alumni groups to gardening clubs and marching bands.

Of course, the number of choices gay people have depends in large part on the size of the gay and lesbian population where they live. For example, in New York City or one of the nation's other major cities, you can choose from a staggering number of social organizations. If you live in a small city or town, the offerings can be limited or nonexistent. But then, you can always hook up with a group elsewhere via the Internet, start a local chapter of an existing organization, or start your own group.

I happen to know a couple of guys who founded a gay running club with exactly two members. They called their group the Kate Smith Running Club, in honor of the late, great—and ample—singer Kate Smith.

Where do gay people vacation?

Gay people go everywhere to vacation, but there are some destinations that are especially popular with gay and lesbian people. These places include Provincetown, which is on the tip of Cape Cod, in Massachusetts; Rehoboth Beach, Delaware; the Pines and Cherry Grove on Fire Island, in New York; Palm Springs and the Russian River, in California; South Beach, in Miami Beach, Florida; and Ft. Lauderdale, also in Florida.

These resort areas offer hotels, restaurants, stores, and bars that are welcoming of or cater to gay and lesbian people. And beyond the physical amenities, these resorts offer something that no other resorts can offer gay people: lots of other gay and lesbian people (especially when there are gay-specific events planned for these places, including parties and gay family weekends). For singles looking for a date or a relationship, these vacation destinations are especially appealing.

When you travel to a popular gay resort area, you know you won't have to worry about being the only gay man or woman on the street or at the beach, no hotel clerk will do a double take when you and your partner check into a room with one bed, and holding hands with your same-sex partner will not likely generate stares. You can relax and be yourself, which for a lot of gay people is an all-too-rare treat.

Of all the gay-friendly resorts, the Pines and Cherry Grove on Fire Island are the gayest. Accessible only by ferry from the eastern end of Long Island, these two small summer communities are almost entirely populated by gay and lesbian people. Of course, heterosexual people are welcome, too.

In addition to traveling to gay resort areas, some gay people who wish to vacation with other gay people go on gay and lesbian cruises, or join group tours that are organized specifically for gay people.

11

Religion

? Is homosexuality a sin and/or immoral?

No, homosexuality is not a sin, and it is not immoral. Of course, not everyone will agree with me, but fortunately, the United States is a nation where morality and religious beliefs are not legislated but are a matter of personal choice—at least so far!

In recent years, these questions of whether or not homosexuality is immoral or sinful have been the subject of great debate. The result has been enormous conflict within the nation's mainstream religions and continuing heated discussion within American society. The following thoughts are from just three of the many people who have offered definitive progay responses to the questions of morality and sin.

Frank Kameny, Gay Rights Pioneer

Frank Kameny, who was fired from his job at the U.S. Army Map Service in 1957 because he was gay, first examined the morality question as part of his fight to get his job back. Kameny pursued his case right up to the U.S. Supreme Court, and in preparing his petition to the Supreme Court in late 1960 he concluded that homosexuality was moral.

"At that time," Kameny explained, "the government put its disqualification of gays under the rubric of immoral conduct, which I objected to. Because under our system, morality is a matter of personal opinion and individual belief on which any American citizen may hold any view he wishes and upon which the government has no power or authority to have any view at all. Besides which, in my view, homosexuality is not only not immoral, but is affirmatively moral. Up until that time nobody else ever said this—as far as I know—in any kind of a formal court pleading."

The Supreme Court refused to hear Kameny's case, and in 1961 he founded a pioneering gay rights organization in Washington, D.C. In part because of Kameny's dogged efforts, the federal government officially stopped excluding homosexuals from government employment in 1975.

Carolyn Mobley, Associate Pastor

Carolyn Mobley, an associate pastor in Houston, Texas, for the Metropolitan Community Church, a Christian church whose membership is primarily gay and lesbian, at first believed that her sexual orientation was sinful. But as a college student, she realized that her sexuality was not sinful but, instead, a "gift from God."

Mobley credits the Reverend Martin Luther King Jr. with helping her come to terms with being a lesbian. She told me, "Dr. King's commitment to disobeying unjust laws had a profound impact on my thinking. I began to question the things that I was told to do: Are they really right? Are they right if I'm told they're right by a person in a position of authority?

"I began to realize that parents could steer you wrong. Teachers could steer you wrong. Preachers, God knows, could steer you wrong. They were all fallible human beings. That really changed my way of looking at myself and the world. And it certainly helped me reevaluate the message I was getting from the church about homosexuality. It made me examine more closely what Scripture had to say about it.

"I continuously read Scripture on my own. I especially reread Romans numerous times. I finally got the picture that God wasn't against homosexuals, and that even Paul, who wrote that passage in Romans about homosexuality and was against homosexuals, was a human being subject to error, just like me. So I thought the man was wrong, period. What he was espousing was inaccurate, and it needed to be challenged. That was what Dr. King was about, challenging error wherever it was found.

"I continued to reinterpret that whole Romans scripture about giving up what was natural for something unnatural, and a light went off in my head. Paul had a point. His argument about doing what was natural really did make sense, but you had to know what was natural for you. It was unnatural for me to have sex with a man, so I decided that I wouldn't do that again. The only natural thing was for me to do what I'd been feeling since Day One in the world. Why would I try to change that? How foolish I'd been. I thought to myself, *Thank you, Paul. I got your message, brother. We're okay.*

"When that light went on in my head, I knew it was from God, that it was my deliverance. God didn't deliver me from my sexuality. God delivered me from guilt and shame and gave me a sense of pride and wholeness that I really needed. My sexuality was a gift from God, and so is everyone's sexuality, no matter how it's oriented. It's a gift to be able to love."

John Shelby Spong, Episcopal Bishop of Newark, New Jersey (Ret.)

Bishop John Shelby Spong, an outspoken supporter of the ordination of gay and lesbian people and the blessing of same-gender relationships, also believes that homosexuality is not a sin. When asked by Parents, Families and Friends of Lesbians and Gays whether, in his opinion, God regards homosexuality as a sin, he answered in writing: "Some argue that since homosexual behavior is 'unnatural,' it is contrary to the order of creation. Behind this pronouncement are stereotypic definitions of masculinity and femininity that reflect the rigid gender categories of patriarchal society.

"There is nothing unnatural about any shared love, even between two people of the same gender, if that experience calls both partners into a fuller state of being. Contemporary research is uncovering new facts that are producing a rising conviction that homosexuality, far from being a sickness, sin, perversion, or unnatural act, is a healthy, natural, and affirming form of human sexuality for some people. Findings indicate that homosexuality is a given fact in the nature of a significant portion of people, and that it is unchangeable.

"Our prejudice rejects people or things outside our understanding. But the God of creation speaks and declares, 'I have looked out on everything I have made and "behold it [is] very good"' [Genesis 1:31]. The word of God in Christ says that we are loved, valued, redeemed, and counted as precious no matter how we might be valued by a prejudiced world."

? Can a gay person become heterosexual through prayer?

A gay person can become heterosexual through prayer just as easily as a heterosexual person can become gay through prayer. In other words—it's impossible. Prayer and/or meditation may help you suppress your God- or nature-given sexual orientation, but prayer will not eliminate these feelings and certainly can't change them.

It may seem harmless to suggest that prayer is the answer for gay people who want to become heterosexual, but as Mary Griffith, who once held Christian fundamentalist beliefs, discovered, it can be deadly. Griffith believed that if Bobby, her teenage gay son, prayed hard enough, he would become heterosexual.

Bobby prayed, all the while fearing that God would punish him for his sexual orientation. He wrote in his diary: "Why did you do this to me, God? Am I going to hell? That's the gnawing question that's always drilling little holes in the back of my mind. Please don't send me to hell. I'm really not that bad, am I? I want to be good. I want to amount to something. I need your seal of approval. If I had that, I would be happy. Life is so cruel and unfair." A year and a half later, at the age of twenty, Bobby jumped off a highway overpass and landed in the path of an eighteen-wheel truck.

In a letter to other gay young people printed in the *San Francisco Examiner,* Mary Griffith later wrote, "I firmly believe—though I did not, back then—that my son Bobby's suicide is the end result of homophobia and ignorance within most Protestant and Catholic churches, and consequently within society, our public schools, our own family.

"Bobby was not drunk, nor did he use drugs. It's just that we could never accept him for who he was—a gay person.

"We hoped God would heal him of being gay. According to God's word, as we were led to understand it, Bobby had to repent or God would damn him to hell and eternal punishment. Blindly, I accepted the idea that it is God's nature to torment and intimidate us.

"That I ever accepted—believed—such depravity of God toward my son or any human being has caused me much remorse and shame. What a travesty of God's love, for children to grow up believing themselves to be evil, with only a slight inclination toward goodness, and that they will remain undeserving of God's love from birth to death.

"Looking back, I realize how depraved it was to instill false guilt in an innocent child's conscience, causing a distorted image of life, God and self, leaving little if any feeling of personal worth.

"Had I viewed my son's life with a pure heart, I would have recognized him as a tender spirit in God's eyes."

The story of Mary Griffith and Bobby Griffith is chronicled in a compelling book, *Prayers for Bobby: A Mother's Coming to Terms with the Suicide of Her Gay Son,* by the late Leroy Aarons (who also founded the National Lesbian and Gay Journalists Association).

? What does the Bible say about gay men and lesbians?

The Bible doesn't say anything about homosexuality as we understand it today. And though the Bible does discuss same-gender sexual relations, it doesn't say all that much about sex between men and says absolutely nothing about sex between women. Among the Bible's 31,173 verses, there are fewer than a dozen that mention sexual acts between men.

I like what Peter J. Gomes, an American Baptist minister and professor of Christian morals at Harvard, had to say in a *New York Times* editorial regarding what is written in the Bible about homosexuality:

> Christians opposed to political and social equality for homosexuals nearly always appeal to the moral injunctions of the Bible, claiming that Scripture is very clear on the matter and citing verses that support their opinion. They accuse others of perverting and distorting texts contrary to their "clear" meaning. They do not, however, necessarily see quite as clear a meaning in biblical passages on economic conduct, the burdens of wealth, and the sin of greed.
>
> Nine biblical citations are customarily invoked as relating to homosexuality. Four (Deuteronomy 23:17, I Kings 14:24, I Kings 22:46, and II Kings 23:7) simply forbid prostitution by men and women. Two others (Leviticus 18:19 – 23 and Leviticus 20:10 – 16) are part of what biblical scholars call the Holiness Code. The code explicitly bans homosexual acts. But it also prohibits eating raw meat, planting two different kinds of seed in the same field and wearing garments with two different kinds of yarn. Tattoos, adultery, and sexual intercourse during a woman's menstrual period are similarly outlawed.
>
> There is no mention of homosexuality in the four Gospels of the New Testament. The moral teachings of Jesus are not concerned with the subject.
>
> Three references from St. Paul are frequently cited (Romans 1:26 – 2:1, I Corinthians 6:9 – 11, and I Timothy 1:10). But St. Paul was concerned with homosexuality only because in Greco-

Roman culture it represented a secular sensuality that was contrary to his Jewish-Christian spiritual idealism. He was against lust and sensuality in anyone, including heterosexuals. To say that homosexuality is bad because homosexuals are tempted to do morally doubtful things is to say that heterosexuality is bad because heterosexuals are likewise tempted. For St. Paul, anyone who puts his or her interest ahead of God's is condemned, a verdict that falls equally upon everyone.

And lest we forget Sodom and Gomorrah, recall that the story is not about sexual perversion and homosexual practice. It is about inhospitality, according to Luke 10:10 – 13, and failure to take care of the poor, according to Ezekiel 16:49 – 50: "Behold, this was the iniquity of thy sister Sodom, pride, fullness of bread, and abundance of idleness was in her and in her daughters, neither did she strengthen the hand of the poor and needy." To suggest that Sodom and Gomorrah is about homosexual sex is an analysis of about as much worth as suggesting that the story of Jonah and the whale is a treatise on fishing.

Gomes goes on to say later in his editorial that "those who speak for the religious right do not speak for all American Christians, and the Bible is not theirs alone to interpret."

The same Bible that the advocates of slavery used to protect their wicked self-interests is the Bible that inspired slaves to revolt and their liberators to action.

The same Bible that the predecessors of [the Reverend Jerry] Falwell and [the Reverend Pat] Robertson used to keep white churches white is the source of the inspiration of the Rev. Martin Luther King, Jr., and the social reformation of the 1960s.

The same Bible that antifeminists use to keep women silent in the churches is the Bible that preaches liberation to captives and says that in Christ there is neither male nor female, slave nor free.

And the same Bible which, on the basis of an archaic social code of ancient Israel and a tortured reading of Paul, is used to condemn all homosexuals and homosexual behavior includes metaphors of redemption, renewal, inclusion and love—principles that invite homosexuals to accept their freedom and responsibility in Christ and demand that their fellow Christians accept them as well.

? What did Jesus have to say about homosexuals or homosexuality?

Nothing. *Rien. Nada.* In any language, it's the same.

? What do different religions say about gay men and lesbians?

The only thing the many different religions agree on about homosexuality is that they don't agree. That goes for different religions as well as different denominations within religions and different religious leaders within the same denomination. But for the sake of bringing a little order to the cacophony of discordant voices within the religious world, here's a general survey of what the major religions in the United States have to say on the subject, drawn, in part, from the *San Francisco Examiner.*

The United Methodists let openly gay people join and do not officially consider homosexuality a sin, but the United Methodists do consider homosexual activity "incompatible with

Christian teaching." Nonetheless, more than 140 "reconciling congregations" have declared themselves to publicly welcome the full participation of gay men and lesbians, and a group of Methodist ministers has declared they will perform same-gender unions.

The Mormon Church (the Church of Jesus Christ of Latter-Day Saints) does not let openly gay people join, considers homosexuality a sin, recommends chastity for homosexuals, and opposes marriage for gay couples.

The Roman Catholic Church permits openly gay people to join, considers homosexuality morally wrong and a sin if practiced, and teaches that any sexual activity outside marriage is wrong. But Roman Catholic bishops in the United States issued a pastoral letter in 1997 advising parents of gay children to love and support their sons and daughters. In their letter the bishops said that homosexual orientation is not freely chosen and that parents must not reject their gay children in a society full of rejection and discrimination.

The letter, which goes on to state that sexual activity between same-gender partners is immoral, urges parents to encourage their children to lead a chaste life. And just in case anyone thought otherwise, the bishops noted that the letter should not be understood "as an endorsement of what some would call 'a homosexual life style.' " And needless to say, the Catholic Church has been extremely vocal in its opposition to extending marriage rights to same-gender couples.

The Baptists officially let openly gay people join and consider homosexuality a sin, but the American Baptists and Southern Baptists differ in their views, and individual churches are autonomous. So although the Southern Baptist Convention may condemn homosexuality as "a manifestation of a depraved nature" and "a perversion of divine standards," one of its member churches, the Pullen Memorial Baptist Church, in Raleigh, North Carolina, held a "blessing of holy union" for two gay men. That church was later ousted from the national convention, and the Southern Baptists subsequently amended their constitution to make it clear that "homosexual behavior" was not to be approved or endorsed by any affiliated church.

The Episcopal Church lets openly gay people join, does not consider homosexuality a sin, and urges congregations to provide dialogues on human sexuality. But the Episcopal Church, which is one of the thirty-seven church provinces within the global Anglican Communion, was rocked by a resolution passed at the once-a-decade Lambeth Conference in 1998. The nearly eight hundred bishops who attended from around the world voted to reject homosexual practice as "incompatible with Scripture." And in more recent years, the ordination of a gay bishop, Gene Robinson, resulted in a bitter debate over the role of gay people in the church.

The Lutherans let openly gay people join, consider homosexuality a sin, and believe that it is not in God's original plan. Presbyterians don't have one voice on this issue except regarding the ordination of gay and lesbian people: The highest court of the Presbyterian Church ruled in November 1992 that an openly gay, sexually active person cannot serve as a minister of any of its 11,500 churches; the ruling nullified the hiring of a gay woman as a copastor of a church in Rochester, New York.

Islam does not accept openly gay people, considers homosexuality one of the worst sins, and encourages homosexuals to change.

Orthodox Jews believe that homosexuality is an abomination. But on the other end of the Jewish spectrum, the Reform and Reconstructionist movements have established special outreach programs for gay and lesbian people and have accepted them publicly into their rabbinical associations. Covering the middle ground of Judaism is the Conservative movement, which has welcomed gay and lesbian people to its congregations but does not allow them to become rabbis.

The best news comes from the Unitarian Universalists and the Buddhists. Buddhists openly welcome gay people, ordain them, don't consider homosexuality a sin, and have no formal teaching policy about gay and lesbian people. The Unitarian Universalist Association, with more than one thousand congregations nationwide, welcomes gay men and women in all church roles. The Unitarians perform holy unions for gay and lesbian couples, Unitarian Universalist churches across the country offer regular sermons and workshops on gay and lesbian issues, and many individual churches host PFLAG meetings and Metropolitan Community Church congregations (a nationwide church whose membership is primarily gay and lesbian).

? Why is there so much antagonism between the Roman Catholic Church and gay people?

The Catholic Church has been extremely harsh in its condemnations of homosexuality and has very actively opposed gay rights efforts. For example, in June 1992 the Vatican sent a memo to the leaders of the nation's more than ten million Roman Catholics reiterating the church's position that homosexuality is an "objective disorder" and insisting that, for the sake of the "common good," U.S. bishops oppose legislation barring discrimination against homosexuals in areas that include adoption, placement of children in foster care, military service, and employment of teachers and athletic coaches. In more recent years, the Vatican has issued statements using the harshest terms in condemning marriage between people of the same gender and urging Roman Catholic politicians to oppose the spread of laws that recognize same-sex couples. The Vatican called the support of such legislation "gravely immoral."

Do all Catholics agree with the official church position on homosexuality?

No matter what their beliefs, not all people agree with all the teachings of their religions, whether those beliefs concern human sexuality, dietary restrictions, or birth control.

For example, I received a letter from a woman whose sister-in-law is a lesbian and was unhappy with what she read in an earlier edition of this book about Catholics and the Catholic Church. She took issue with the impression she believes I had left that all Catholics think one way about gay and lesbian people. She wrote: "Your emphasis may lead to a conclusion that Catholics gain nothing from their religion but homophobia and guilt. I hate to generalize, so I'll simply observe that this isn't true for me.

"What I get from my religious advisors is almost the opposite. The very word 'Catholic' means accepting everyone. I've learned at church that God doesn't make junk, and this helps me pay no heed to people who would deny human or social rights to gays and lesbians. . . .

"You accurately state that the Church does require gay Catholics to be celibate, much as it requires us not to use birth control (although in practice, both teachings are often honored in the breach). It does not require that we vote in any particular way. . . .

"It would be a shame if anyone concluded they shouldn't come out to a sympathetic friend because the friend is Catholic. Some gay people may need all the friends they can get. I do, too, and some of them are gay."

Is the Catholic Church the only religious group that has actively opposed the rights of gay people?

Hardly. Many fundamentalist religious organizations and leaders have for years taken a very active role in opposing any efforts to extend equal rights to gay people, and some have worked hard at demonizing gay people as a group set on the destruction of the American family.

Have organized religions always opposed homosexuality?

According to the historian John Boswell, in his book *Christianity, Social Tolerance, and Homosexuality,* up until the end of the twelfth century Christian moral theology treated homosexuality "as, at worst, comparable to heterosexual fornication but more often remained silent on the issue." But then, on the heels of a diatribe from Saint Thomas Aquinas, the church began to view homosexuals as both unnatural and dangerous.

Are there organizations and places of worship specifically for gay people who are religious?

There are organizations all across the country specifically for gay and lesbian people who are Catholic, Jewish, Episcopal, Muslim, Lutheran, ... You name it, there's an organization.

(An online search will quickly get you to the religious organization of your choosing.)

Also, most major cities have a gay synagogue. In addition, the Metropolitan Community Church, whose membership is primarily gay and lesbian, has hundreds of congregations in the United States and around the world.

Can openly gay people become religious leaders?

Yes, but it depends upon the religion, denomination, and/or individual congregation. Of course, there are already many religious leaders serving in churches, synagogues, and even mosques around the country who are gay, but because most of them are compelled to keep their sexual orientation a secret, no one knows how many.

Haven't some religious institutions and leaders been involved in fighting for equal rights for gay people?

Some religious institutions and members of the clergy have been very actively involved in supporting equal rights for gay people.

Perhaps the earliest example of support from religious leaders came in 1965, when a group of liberal ministers in San Francisco, along with local gay rights activists, staged the first major public gay and lesbian fund-raising event in that city for a new organization called the Council on Religion and the Homosexual.

The Unitarian Universalists were also gay rights pioneers. In 1970 they called for an end to discrimination against gay and lesbian people in the denomination and in society, declaring that private consensual sexual behavior was a private matter.

? What can you say to religious people who say about gay people, "Love the sinner, but hate the sin"?

I would tell you what I'd *really* like to say, but that would not be very constructive, nor would it be terribly Christian. So I'll tell you what I usually say when faced with that comment: "Thank you, but I can live without that kind of love."

I think the "love the sinner, hate the sin" philosophy is a convenient way for Christian people who condemn homosexuality to reconcile their feelings about gay men and women. They can feel good about loving the "sinner" and also feel good about not compromising their religious beliefs by proclaiming their hatred for the "sin."

The problem with this construct is that it assumes you can separate the alleged sin from the alleged sinner. The fact is, the "sin," my sexual orientation and how I choose to express it, is as much a part of me, the "sinner," as my skin, my eye color, or the gray matter between my ears. So if you hate something as fundamental to me as my skin, then you necessarily hate me, too. It's hard to imagine well-meaning people of faith feeling very good about *that!*

12

Discrimination and Antigay Violence

? How are gay people discriminated against?

Gay and lesbian people are discriminated against in many different ways. People have, for example, been fired from their jobs, evicted from their apartments, and denied custody of their children. Gay people are routinely discharged from the military. Gay student groups have been refused official recognition by high schools and universities. Gay boys are not permitted to join the Boy Scouts. And gay and lesbian couples, no matter how many years they have been together, are denied the same protections given to straight married couples in all but a handful of states in the United States.

But usually the discrimination experienced by gay people isn't nearly so obvious as getting fired. More typical (and insidious) is a landlord who won't rent to two "single" men (only married couples) or a boss who never follows through on a promised job promotion.

? Aren't there laws that prohibit discrimination against gay people?

There are, but the laws don't apply everywhere, and they're not uniform in their protections. But even if gay people were granted full equal rights and broad legal protections from discrimination, such rights and protections would not eliminate discrimination.

As we know from hard-won civil rights protections put in place during the 1960s to protect African Americans from discrimination, legal protections did not bring an automatic end to racism and discrimination. The legal protections were in some ways just a start. A law protecting you from discrimination may give you legal recourse if you're the target of discrimination, but it does not erase prejudice from people's hearts. That kind of social and personal change requires much effort over a long period of time.

If you would like to know what, if any, laws protect gay people from discrimination where you live, visit the Web site for Lambda Legal (www.lambdalegal.com), a national organization that is, by its own description "committed to achieving full recognition of the civil rights of lesbians, gay men, bisexuals, transgender people and those with HIV through impact litigation, education and public policy work."

? How are gay and lesbian people harassed?

Harassment of gay and lesbian people ranges from name-calling and spray-painting antigay epithets on the houses of gay and lesbian people to slashing tires on cars parked outside gay bars. Harassment is particularly common among high school and even middle school students.

All too often, antigay incidents go well beyond name-calling to death threats, beatings, and even murder.

Are gay people really murdered because they're gay?

Yes. For example, in 2003, six men and women were killed in the United States because of their sexual orientation. (That was a year in which there were 1,430 reported hate crimes based on sexual orientation.)

Perhaps the most widely publicized gay murder case was the 1998 killing of Matthew Shepard, a University of Wyoming student who was kidnapped, robbed, pistol-whipped, and left tied to a fence for eighteen hours in near-freezing temperatures. His death five days later led to outrage across the country and a call for a national hate-crime law that would include crimes based on sexual orientation. In the end, no such laws were passed.

The playwright Moisés Kaufman created a play called *The Laramie Project,* which chronicles the life of the town of Laramie, Wyoming, in the year following the Matthew Shepard murder. HBO produced a 2002 film based on the play.

Why do people dislike, hate, discriminate against, harass, and attack gay men and lesbians?

Some do so because they believe homosexuality is sinful and immoral or that gay people are child molesters, disease carriers, and/or mentally ill. Others believe that homosexuality is contrary to good moral values and threatens to destroy the

American family. (I've never heard a good explanation of exactly *how* gay people are a threat to the American family.)

The University of California research psychologist Dr. Gregory M. Herek, the author of *Hate Crimes: Confronting Violence Against Lesbians and Gay Men,* states that for most people who are biased against gay people, homosexuals "stand as a proxy for all that is evil . . . such people see hating gay men and lesbians as a litmus test for being a moral person."

Other psychologists who have studied antigay bias say it results from a combination of fear and self-righteousness in which gay people are perceived as contemptible threats to the moral universe. These antigay feelings are often supported by religious institutions that consider homosexuality to be sinful.

Young people in particular are often motivated in their verbal or physical attacks on gay people by a desire to be a part of the crowd or to gain approval of their peers or family. And some men are motivated by fear of their own homosexual feelings. Though Dr. Herek thinks that this explanation is used more often than is the case, "it does apply to some men who will attack gays as a way of denying unacceptable aspects of their personalities."

? Is antigay violence a new problem or a big problem?

As I discovered when I began interviewing older gay people for my history book, antigay violence is nothing new. Barbara Gittings, an early gay rights activist, recalled an incident in the 1950s at a gay bar in New York City: "I was with my friend Pinky, who got friendly with a couple of uniformed guys, Marines, I believe. They were sitting and talking with us. When the four of us left the bar, out came the brass knuckles and they proceeded to rip up Pinky's face. They said to me, 'We aren't touching you, Sonny, because you wear glasses.'

"It was terrifying, and there was not a damn thing I could do until they had finished their dirty work and left. Then I helped Pinky up and got him to a hospital. He had thirteen stitches in his nose. I guess in my innocence I hadn't thought people could be so hateful and violent toward us."

Several early activists I spoke with said that after such experiences they were reluctant to call the police because more often than not the police wouldn't do anything, and, on occasion, the police were the ones who had administered the beatings.

In recent years, public authorities have taken the issue of antigay violence more seriously, in part spurred on by government reports that concluded that gay people are the most frequent victims of hate-motivated violence.

? Are there organizations that combat antigay violence?

Yes, and most are members of the National Coalition of Anti-Violence Programs (www.ncavp.org). NCAVP is an umbrella organization for lesbian, gay, bisexual, and transgender victim-advocacy and documentation programs throughout the United States.

These programs and organizations typically work in their cities and states to combat antigay violence. They do this in a number of ways, including educating police departments about gay and lesbian people and the problem of antigay violence and working with victims and witnesses to gather information they would otherwise be reluctant to convey directly to the police. Some organizations also send speakers into local high schools to educate students about gay and lesbian people, with the goal of heading off antigay violence.

NCAVP issues an annual report on antigay violence, and the organization, along with many of the local antiviolence groups, works at the state and national levels to lobby for hate-crimes laws that include crimes based on sexual orientation.

? What are hate-crimes laws, and how can these prevent antigay violence?

Hate-crimes laws generally increase penalties for crimes motivated by prejudice. In other words, someone who assaults a Jewish man because he's Jewish could be charged with a hate crime in addition to being charged with assault and battery—as long as that crime was committed in a state that has hate-crimes laws on the books.

Not everyone agrees that hate-crimes laws make any difference. Some people argue that such laws are an important tool in prosecuting and deterring hate crimes, and others believe that such laws have no impact or restrict political speech.

? How can someone report antigay violence?

The first thing to do is to call the police and, if need be, call for emergency medical assistance. You should also call your local gay antiviolence organization to report the incident. To find the group nearest to you and/or to get more information on antigay violence (and gay domestic violence), visit the Web site for the National Coalition of Anti-Violence Programs (www.ncavp.org).

? What should you do if you're gay and being harassed?

It depends upon the circumstances. If you're a middle school or high school student and you're comfortable talking to your parents, tell them what's going on and ask them to talk to the school's principal. Or if you're not comfortable talking to your parents, you can talk to your school guidance counselor. (But make sure you can count on the counselor to keep your talk confidential.)

Or, if there's a gay-straight alliance at your school, you can talk to the group's adviser and ask the adviser to speak to the principal. You could also talk to the principal yourself. If the principal or school administrators fail to respond, or you're afraid to talk to the principal or school authorities or fear they won't keep your confidence, contact a local or national gay organization to enlist their help. (See the "Resources" section at the back of this book for contact information.)

If the problem occurs at work and you can speak to your boss or human-resources department about it without fear of losing your job, then tell them what's going on. If you're in a job where you can't talk to those in charge, I recommend contacting the appropriate gay organization to get advice on how to handle your specific circumstances.

Sometimes the best thing to do is to call the police, which is what my then-partner and I did when we were threatened by our neighbor in the San Francisco (San Francisco!) apartment house where we lived. Our neighbor and his friends, all employees of a federal security agency, had had a lot too much to drink and decided to threaten to shoot the "fags" upstairs with their AK-47 assault rifles.

We had no way of knowing if these guys were really armed,

but we didn't think it was worth taking any chances, so we called the police. It was a terrifying experience, which cost us several sleepless nights and cost our neighbor his apartment. Our landlord evicted him within weeks of the incident.

? What should you do if you're gay and you've been discriminated against?

If you live in a place where there are no laws protecting gay people from discrimination, you may have no recourse. If there are such laws, you may be able to fight back, but discrimination is tough to prove. I suggest contacting a local or national gay rights or legal organization to get advice on what to do. See the "Resources" section at the back of this book for a list of organizations.

? Do gay people discriminate?

As I've said many times by now, gay people are like everyone else. So don't think that just because many gay men and women know what it's like to be discriminated against, we're not fully capable of turning around and doing the same to others, whether we discriminate on the basis of skin color, physical appearance, or style of dress.

I like the observation made by Martin Block, an early member of the Mattachine Society, a gay rights group founded in 1950: "Any time there was a proposal to do something public, people argued, 'Well, I don't want those drag queens coming' or 'I don't want that one coming' or 'Isn't she outrageous with her constant swish?'

"I'm not saying that drag queens were not welcome. I'm saying that they were not welcome by *everybody.* In every gay movement there has always been a schism. Some people don't want anyone who sticks his little pinkie out, and some people don't want anyone who doesn't stick his little pinkie out. None of us is without bias. And I am delighted to say that I am full of bias myself, but my bias is mostly against stupidity."

13

Movies, Television, and Print Media

? Are gay people portrayed accurately in the movies?

Over the years gay and lesbian people—individually, through organized protests, and through the Gay and Lesbian Alliance Against Defamation (GLAAD; www.glaad.org) have complained plenty about how gay people have been portrayed in mainstream Hollywood-produced movies. And with good reason.

Until recent years, almost without exception gay and lesbian people have been portrayed in mainstream films as murderers, twisted villains, victims, or wimps. And even when there weren't homicidal or suicidal gay characters onscreen, it was difficult to get through a movie without someone making an anti-gay joke or using offensive words like "fag" and "dyke." All this is thoroughly documented by the late film historian Vito Russo in his book *The Celluloid Closet: Homosexuality in the Movies*.

Gay men and lesbians aren't the only group of people to suffer at the hands of filmmakers. Every minority group—ethnic, racial, religious, or otherwise—has been portrayed negatively at one time or another. The difference is that when it comes to gay and lesbian people, for most of Hollywood's history there has rarely been any attempt to portray them in a realistic and balanced manner.

Though positive gay and lesbian characters are still not commonplace in Hollywood-produced movies, they've turned up in several films, including Paul Rudnick's hilarious *In and Out*, *My Best Friend's Wedding*, *The Object of My Affection*, and *As Good As It Gets*.

? But aren't there other movies where gay men and lesbians come off pretty well?

Yes, but they've been produced independently for theatrical release, or you'll find them on HBO or other cable stations. Some of these films include *Angels in America; Gods and Monsters; The Opposite of Sex; The Wedding Banquet; The Adventures of Priscilla, Queen of the Desert; Go Fish; When Night Is Falling; French Twist*; and *All Over Me*.

? Have gay people been portrayed accurately on television?

When I was a kid growing up in the 1960s, *Lost in Space* was my favorite television show. It's a space-age *Swiss Family Robinson* story, complete with a robot and an evil stowaway, Dr. Smith. When I saw an episode not long ago, I was stunned to realize that Dr. Smith was clearly played as a stereotypical gay man: effeminate, timid, and physically weak. He also happened to be duplicitous, scheming, and irredeemably narcissistic. Week after week he put the lives of the other characters at risk as he sought to enrich himself, fill his stomach, or find his way back to Earth. Not exactly a fine role model.

For most of its history, television simply ignored gay men and women, except for the occasional Dr. Smith-style homosexual or Miss Hathaway lesbian (on *The Beverly Hillbillies*). In later years, homosexuality was treated as a "special issue," and when AIDS came along, gay men with AIDS began showing up as single-episode guests.

Gay characters first started appearing on network television shows in the early 1970s, including an episode of the *Mary Tyler Moore Show.* And the first regularly appearing gay character—played by Billy Crystal—hit the airwaves in the late 1970s on ABC's *Soap*.

But in general, it wasn't until the 1990s that gay men and women were simply absorbed into a script without much of a fuss. And by the end of the century, more than twenty supporting gay and lesbian characters were scattered throughout the prime-time television schedule. In 1998, *Will and Grace*, a show that features a gay man and his female heterosexual best friend, made its debut and quickly became one of the most popular situation comedies on broadcast television.

Daytime television has also had its gay moments and characters, perhaps most notably in 2000. That was the year fans of *All My Children* witnessed the coming out of Bianca (played by Eden Riegel), daughter of the very heterosexual Erica Kane (played by Susan Lucci).

The biggest fuss during the 1990s over a gay character involved the coming out of Ellen Morgan, played by the comedienne Ellen DeGeneres, who came out along with her television character (and landed on the cover of *Time* magazine).

The 1997 coming-out episode of *Ellen* drew an audience of more than forty million viewers, including many gay and lesbian people who attended fund-raising viewing parties. I attended one of those parties, and I thought the episode was wonderfully written and very funny. A year later, ABC canceled *Ellen*, citing declining ratings. Ellen DeGeneres got the last laugh and came back a few years later with a very successful syndicated daytime television talk show.

In more recent years gay people have been most visible on a regular basis on cable television, including Bravo's *Queer Eye for the Straight Guy* (a straight-guy makeover show hosted by five gay guys), Showtime's *Queer as Folk* (a drama about a group of gay men) and *The L Word* (a drama about a group of lesbian friends), and HBO's *Six Feet Under*, which includes among its characters a gay male couple who are closer to the real thing than anything else I've seen on television.

For the most current information regarding gay people on television, visit GLAAD's Web site (www.glaad.org).

? Why do the people who advertise on television sometimes object to gay characters or themes on TV?

Advertisers traditionally avoid being associated with any controversial topic, particularly homosexuality. They fear turning off potential customers and don't want to invite the wrath of antigay activists through, for example, product boycotts. Because of this fear, advertisers sometimes pull their sponsorship from shows they object to. And it's not just television. Gay and lesbian publications have fought hard to get and retain advertisers, which has proven challenging during the more conservative years of the new century.

For more on advertising and the gay market, visit the Web site for the Commercial Closet (www.commercialcloset.org).

Why do gay people have their own magazines and newspapers? When did the first of these publications appear?

Gay and lesbian publications offer two things that mass-market, mainstream publications can't. First, they provide gay and lesbian readers with the kind of in-depth news and information they want about issues that concern them and that they aren't likely to find anywhere else. Second, they serve advertisers trying to reach the gay and lesbian market.

The very first publication intended for a same-sex audience was *Vice Versa,* which made its debut in 1947. But only a handful of people ever saw the nine issues that were published by Lisa Ben, a Hollywood secretary, who wrote the newsletter on her office typewriter. She used five pieces of carbon paper and typed each issue of the newsletter through twice, producing a total of ten copies, which she distributed to her friends.

The first gay and lesbian magazines were published in the 1950s by the earliest of the gay organizations and included *ONE, The Ladder,* and the *Mattachine Review.* Today there are more than ten national gay and lesbian magazines—news, travel, general interest—and hundreds of local and regional newspapers and magazines.

What did newspapers and magazines say about gay people in the old days—the 1950s and 1960s?

When the first gay and lesbian magazines were published in the 1950s, they were just about the only places where gay and lesbian people could read *anything* about themselves that wasn't awful. On the rare occasions when the mainstream press chose to write about gay people, the stories were uniformly negative. Here are some typical 1950s headlines drawn from newspapers from around the country: "Nest of Perverts Raided," "How L.A. Handles Its 150,000 Perverts," "Great Civilizations Plagued by Deviates," and "Pervert Colony Uncovered in Simpson Slaying Probe."

Newspapers and magazines published articles about gay people with increasing frequency through the 1960s and 1970s, much of it biased and/or hostile. One of my favorite examples comes from an unsigned essay in the January 21, 1966, issue of *Time* magazine.

The essay, entitled "The Homosexual in America," stated, "For many a woman with a busy or absent husband, the presentable homosexual is in demand as an escort—witty, pretty, catty, and no problem to keep at arm's length.... The once widespread view that homosexuality is caused by heredity, or some derangement of hormones, has been generally discarded. The consensus is that it is caused psychically, through a disabling fear of the opposite sex."

The essay noted that both male and female homosexuality were "essentially a case of arrested development, a failure of learning, a refusal to accept the full responsibilities of life. This is no more apparent than in the pathetic pseudo marriages in which many homosexuals act out conventional roles—wearing wedding rings, calling themselves 'he' and 'she.' "

The *Time* essayist saved the best for last: "[Homosexuality] is a pathetic little second-rate substitute for reality, a pitiable flight from life. As such it deserves fairness, compassion, understanding and when possible, treatment. But it deserves no encouragement, no glamorization, no rationalization, no fake status as minority martyrdom, no sophistry about simple differences in taste—and above all, no pretense that it is anything but a pernicious sickness."

Today, many mainstream publications are doing a fine job of accurately reporting major gay and lesbian stories, but no matter how good they get, mass-market newspapers and magazines can't offer gay and lesbian readers and advertisers what local and national special-market publications can.

When did newspapers first start publishing gay commitment-ceremony and wedding announcements?

In November 1990, the *Everett Herald,* in Everett, Washington, published the first same-sex commitment-ceremony announcement.

My hometown newspaper, the *New York Times,* first began publishing such announcements on September 1, 2002. The first same-sex pair featured by the *New York Times* was Daniel Gross and Steven Goldstein. Several hundred mainstream newspapers now publish same-sex-ceremony announcements.

Are there gay newspaper and television reporters?

Plenty, which has led in no small part to a quiet revolution since the 1980s in reporting on gay and lesbian people and issues. (The late Randy Shilts, the author of the 1987 bestseller *And the Band Played On,* was the first openly gay journalist to gain national stature.)

As more and more journalists, television reporters, editors, and producers have gone public with their sexual orientation, they have helped their news organizations—from newspapers and magazines to broadcast television and cable—more accurately report on gay and lesbian people and issues.

For more information, visit the Web site for the National Lesbian and Gay Journalists Association (www.nlgja.org).

? Do gay people have their own books?

You're holding one, although not everyone who reads this book is gay.

The number of books published each year for gay and lesbian people has grown dramatically since the 1970s, and these days you can find books for gay people written on every imaginable topic—from young-adult novels (Alex Sanchez has written some of my favorites) and sci-fi mysteries, to history, to relationship-advice books.

Some bookstores—both independents and national chains—have special (although often pitifully stocked) gay and lesbian sections. And there are also independent bookstores in several cities that specialize in books of interest to gay, lesbian, bisexual, and transgender people. The first of these bookstores, the Oscar Wilde Memorial Bookshop, opened in 1967 in New York City's Greenwich Village.

14

Sports

? Why don't gay men like sports?

Okay, I admit it: I don't like competitive sports and couldn't care less which baseball or football team is in first place. And I could never understand why anyone would want to waste a sunny (or rainy, for that matter) Saturday or Sunday afternoon glued to the television watching his or her favorite sports team.

Add to these facts my pathetic performance on the ball field at summer camp, and I should have known I was gay, right? But what about one of my gay male friends, who flies from city to city to follow his favorite football team and is an avid triathlete? And how do you explain the thousands of gay men who participate in the Gay Games (see "What are the Gay Games?" later in this chapter), not to mention the many closeted gay male professional athletes?

The fact is, lots of men are good at and/or like sports, and that includes lots of gay men. And plenty of men are bad at and/or don't like sports, and that includes plenty of straight guys.

Are all women athletes and physical-education teachers lesbians?

One of the classic stereotypes about lesbians is that they're all good athletes. Indeed, there are women athletes and physical-education teachers who are lesbians, but there are also plenty of lesbians like my friend Linda, who can't throw a ball or swing a golf club to save her life. And, of course, there are plenty of women athletes and physical-education teachers who are heterosexual.

According to Dr. Dee Mosbacher, a psychiatrist who produced a documentary on homophobia and women in sports, the question isn't how many lesbians are in sports, but why some people are playing into the public's fear of homosexuality and accusing women in sports of being lesbians.

"The charge of lesbianism," explained Dr. Mosbacher, "is used for several reasons. For example, when recruiting women athletes for college, some coaches have tried to attract certain women by suggesting that the coach at a competing school is a lesbian. And the charge of lesbianism has also been used to discourage or avoid hiring female coaches. As women's sports have become significantly more lucrative in recent years, and more men have been competing for coaching jobs, we've seen an increase in this kind of accusation against women coaches."

What are the Gay Games?

Well, they were originally called the Gay Olympics, but the U.S. Olympic Committee, which by an act of Congress owns the word *Olympic*, brought a lawsuit prior to the first Gay Games and succeeded in preventing the event's organizers from using the word. And this was despite the fact that there had been many other legally unquestioned "Olympics" for all kinds of things, including Olympics for dogs, frogs, and hamburger chefs.

The first International Gay Athletic Games were held from August 29 through September 5, 1982, in San Francisco. More than thirteen hundred athletes from fifteen countries participated. Dr. Tom Waddell, a 1968 U.S. Olympic decathlete, founded the Gay Games (and also helped organize the famous protest by black U.S. athletes at the 1968 Summer Olympics in Mexico City).

The Gay Games are held every four years in cities around the world. (Eleven thousand athletes from seventy countries attended the 2002 Gay Games in Sydney, Australia.) The purpose of the Gay Games, according to a Gay Games spokesperson, is to "hold a true Olympic event, open to all participants, whose goal is to do their personal best. The event is sponsored by the lesbian and gay community to celebrate lesbians and gay men and promote our self-esteem, pride, and dignity."

? Are there openly gay star athletes?

Very few professional athletes—star or otherwise—have come out of the closet during or after their careers. The list of professional athletes who have come out is short and includes tennis champion Martina Navratilova; four-time Olympic gold-medal diver Greg Louganis; 1996 U.S. figure-skating champion Rudy Galindo (who was never really *in* the closet); former San Francisco 49ers running back Dave Kopay; golfer Muffin Spencer-Devlin; former Oakland A's outfielder Glenn Burke; Wimbledon tennis champion Conchita Martinez; swimmer Bruce Hayes, who won a gold medal at the 1984 summer

Olympics in the 800-meter freestyle relay and seven gold medals at the 1990 Gay Games; Australian rugby player Ian Roberts, who came out in 1994 while he was still an active competitor; tennis star Billie Jean King; and Esera Tuaolo, who played for nine years as a defensive lineman in the NFL.

? Who was the first gay professional athlete to go public?

Former San Francisco 49ers running back Dave Kopay came out publicly in 1975 and went on to write a bestselling book about his life called *The David Kopay Story*.

Kopay went public about his sexual orientation soon after retiring from professional football. He had hoped to land a coaching job on the college level. But after he came out he couldn't find anyone willing to hire him at any level, so he went to work at his uncle's floor-covering store in Hollywood, California.

? Are gay athletes afraid of the consequences if they come out? Is that why most of them hide their sexual orientation?

Professional athletes who are gay fear risking their careers and their safety, as well as potentially lucrative product endorsements, should their homosexuality become public knowledge.

? What about the nonprofessionals, like high school and college athletes? Are they also afraid?

Yes, they're afraid, which is why nearly all gay and lesbian high school and college athletes keep their sexual orientation a secret. Young female athletes are more likely to come out and find acceptance than young male athletes, but I hasten to add that openly gay high school and college athletes, male or female, remain a relatively rare exception.

The National Collegiate Athletic Association (NCAA) added sexual orientation to its nondiscrimination policy for college athletic programs in 2002. And the *NCAA News,* the NCAA's official publication, has begun to explore the issue of gay athletes in its articles and editorials. That's a good start, but there's a very long way to go before gay student athletes can be themselves without fear of being ostracized, verbally abused, physically harmed, and/or pushed off their teams.

15

Education

? What do young people learn about homosexuality in school (K–12)?

Students learn plenty about homosexuality in school, almost all of it informally and nearly all of it bad. The lessons begin in the elementary school cafeteria when one child calls another "fag," continue through middle school, where "Don't be so gay" is the all-around put-down of choice, and are completed in high school when a group of students decides to torment a theater teacher they think is gay.

Formal education about homosexuality is more remarkable for what is *not* said than for what *is* said, because with few exceptions, almost nothing is said. School curricula are virtually devoid of gay subjects. The decades-long history of the gay civil rights movement doesn't come up in social-studies lessons that include discussions about women's rights and black civil rights.

Historical and contemporary figures—authors, artists, politicians, and so on—who are gay are rarely if ever identified as such. High school textbooks mention not a word about gay and lesbian anything. And if a school district has an official policy about teaching gay and lesbian issues, that policy is more often than not to forbid the mention of gay and lesbian people and issues in any positive context.

There are, however, exceptions. Several states, as well as the District of Columbia, have policies that protect gay, lesbian, bisexual, and transgender students and staff from discrimination and harassment. And some of the nation's largest school districts provide workshops for teachers on gay, lesbian, bisexual, and transgender youth issues, and have incorporated lessons on the lives and accomplishments of gay and lesbian people into the curriculum.

The various national education organizations, including the two largest teachers' unions, have also been supportive of educating students about gay and lesbian people, helping teachers learn how to talk about homosexuality, and making counseling available to gay and lesbian teens. In general, these efforts have been very slow to trickle down to the local level, where the majority of individual school boards are politically conservative.

? Can you give some examples of schools where kids learn about gay people in a positive way?

However gloomy I might sound on this subject, there are definitely good things to report in some school districts and at individual schools. For example, some schools invite special guests (like me) to speak about gay and lesbian issues. Some have shown educational documentaries, including *It's Elementary: Talking About Gay Issues in School,* and *Out of the Past.* Some have public bulletin boards where news stories about gay issues are posted. Some school libraries have books about the subject (like *What If Someone I Know Is Gay?,* my question-and-answer book for kids ages ten and up). And some individual teachers have included gay and lesbian issues in their regular lessons, usually in the context of English, health, or civics classes.

For example, Chris Lord, who teaches sixth-grade American history and seventh-grade civics at a private school in Annapolis, Maryland, includes gay and lesbian issues when he thinks it's appropriate: "We do a civil rights movement unit, and it's most appropriate to use something current, like the gay rights movement."

Lord said that more often than not, the subject comes up as a natural part of class discussions. "For example," he told me, "in my sixth-grade class, I questioned someone's use of the word "redneck." Then we went through a lot of the put-down words people use, and the kids locked on to the word "faggot." That led to a thirty-five minute discussion."

One reason students are comfortable discussing gay issues in his class, Lord thinks, is that he usually volunteers the fact that he has a gay father. Lord told me, "On the wall next to my desk, I have a picture of my dad and his partner." Lord also maintains a bulletin board in his class where news items about gay issues are posted.

? Are there clubs or organizations for gay kids at middle schools and high schools?

Yes, hundreds of them, mostly gay-straight alliances (GSAs), and mostly at high schools. The first high school GSA was started in 1991 at the Concord Academy, a private high school in Concord, Massachusetts. The goal of this first group, as it is with all GSAs, is to provide a supportive and safe forum for open discussion between gay and nongay students about the issues that gay, lesbian, bisexual, and transgender students face in school, with their families, and within their communities. GSAs are open to all students, and no student has to identify his or her sexual orientation. (Visit www.glsen.org for information on which schools have GSAs.)

? Are there any organizations working with schools to make things better for gay students and to promote a better understanding of gay issues?

Yes. Since its start in the early 1990s, the Gay, Lesbian and Straight Education Network (GLSEN) has become a driving force in changing what students are taught about homosexuality and how gay, lesbian, bisexual, and transgender students are treated.

GLSEN works as an advocate with mainstream education organizations, including the two largest national teachers' unions and the National School Board Association, on issues ranging from the implementation of nondiscrimination policies that specifically mention sexual orientation to the provision of training workshops for school staff on the issues faced by gay youth. For more information on GLSEN, visit their Web site (www.glsen.org).

? What objections do people have to teaching students about homosexuality?

Teaching students about anything related to gay people or gay life will turn them gay and lead to the destruction of the American way of life.

How's that for a start?

But usually the comments are not nearly that tame and are expressed by an enraged parent at the top of his or her lungs at a school-board meeting. For example: "You are trying to recruit our children!" "You want to teach little children about a sick and perverted lifestyle!" "God created Adam and Eve, not Adam and Steve!" Well, you get the picture.

I don't mean to sound like a broken record, but gay people don't recruit straight kids to become gay (a losing proposition at any rate), we don't as a rule have a "perverted lifestyle" (we don't as a rule have any uniform lifestyle), and many people, including significant numbers of religious leaders, believe that God created gay people just as he created all other people and loves them just the same (although one wonders why God, if there is a God, hasn't given up on humanity in general by now).

When I hear the objections people make, it only confirms for me that change is essential. If we don't do something different than we've done in the past in terms of educating kids about gay people and gay life, we're doomed to bestow on the next generation the old stereotypes, archaic myths, and ancient fears that have plagued our own.

? Are there schools especially for gay and lesbian kids?

There is at least one high school for gay, lesbian, bisexual, and transgender students: the Harvey Milk School, in New York City. It is a small, specialized alternative school for students who, for any number of reasons, are having difficulty attending mainstream high schools.

The Harvey Milk School opened in 1985. It is part of the New York City public school system and is run by the Hetrick-

Martin Institute, a nonprofit organization that provides counseling and other services to gay, lesbian, bisexual, and transgender youth. (For more information on the Hetrick-Martin Institute, visit their Web site: www.hmi.org.)

The students who attend Harvey Milk are kids who had trouble surviving at their local public high schools and requested admission to the alternative school. These are kids who were teased about the way they acted or the way they dressed and were in some cases abused and beaten.

The purpose of the Harvey Milk School is to reintegrate these students into traditional high schools or, failing that, to provide them with a safe place where they can come to terms with their lives and get their high school diplomas.

? Are there openly gay and lesbian schoolteachers?

At the college level there are many, at least compared with how many there were in the late 1970s, when I was in college and there were virtually none. (But don't expect to find openly gay teachers at the colleges and universities run by conservative religious institutions.)

In grades K–12 there are comparatively few openly gay teachers, even in places where gay teachers are protected by law from discrimination. The primary reason for this situation is persistent societal prejudice regarding gay people working with children. And for this reason, gay teachers who work with children are often fearful that if their sexual orientation becomes known their jobs could be in jeopardy, laws or no laws.

Do gay teachers influence or teach their students to be gay? Are gay teachers bad role models?

As you may recall, I address this question in chapter 8, "Work and the Military." But it bears repeating that homosexual teachers can't influence their students to become homosexual any more than heterosexual teachers can influence their students to become heterosexual. Openly gay teachers *can,* however, be positive role models for all kids, just the same as their straight colleagues.

Meet Jim. Jim is a high school teacher in New York City. He is gay and makes no effort to hide his sexual orientation, nor does he make any effort to hide his frustration with parents who object to his presence in the classroom.

Jim told me, "First of all, I don't talk about being gay all the time. But if it comes up, I'm not gonna lie about it. And when it's in the news, the kids wanna talk about it. They have questions. Should I tell them to go read a book because I'm not allowed to talk about it, because if I talk about it they'll wanna be gay like me? These parents need to get an education.

"Look, telling the truth about homosexuals doesn't hurt anyone. I'm educating the straight kids by letting them see a teacher who happens to be gay and does a good job. And the gay and lesbian kids get to see that you can be honest about who you are and have a life and a good career."

Do Jim and other openly gay teachers, just by their example, encourage more gay and lesbian young people to be open about their lives? There's every reason to believe that this is the case. And what's bad about that? Should we encourage gay kids to hide or pretend they're straight? What does that accomplish?

Are there college courses about gay people or gay civil rights history?

As of 2005, more than 150 colleges and universities offered some courses in gay and lesbian studies, with course titles that included "Sexual Orientation and the Law," "Gay and Lesbian Issues in the Workplace," "Selected Issues in Human Sexuality," "Studies in Gay and Bisexual Literature," and "Gay Literature and Film."

In addition to offering courses, nearly thirty colleges recognize a major, minor, or concentration in the field of gay studies. These schools include Allegheny College, in Pennsylvania; Brown University, in Rhode Island; Duke University, in North Carolina; Rice University, in Houston; San Francisco State University; City University of New York; the University of Chicago; the University of Iowa at Iowa City; the University of Wisconsin at Milwaukee; and Yale University, in Connecticut.

Besides formal courses, college students may first hear about homosexuality during orientation—when all kinds of things are discussed, from where to find a good pizza to how to prevent the spread of sexually transmitted diseases. Gay and lesbian issues also come up in a variety of courses, from English literature to history.

Are there colleges and universities that are more or less welcoming of gay students?

If you're gay and don't want to hide that fact, I suggest looking very carefully at prospective schools before you commit your time and money to a place that doesn't want you, is going to make your life miserable, or will throw you out if you're found out.

That's because although many schools are supportive of and embrace their gay and lesbian students (at least one hundred colleges and universities maintain centers that provide support services for gay, lesbian, bisexual, and transgender students), plenty of others don't.

Catholic universities and other schools run by conservative religious institutions do not welcome discussion about gay issues, and gay students are unlikely even to find a place on campus where they can meet. And at the most conservative schools, that's the least of it.

? Are women's colleges all lesbian?

I decided to put this question to a lesbian friend who graduated not very long ago from a prestigious all-women's college. Here's her answer: "Unfortunately, no. I don't even think it's disproportionate."

That said, some schools—exclusively female or coed—give the impression of having more gay and lesbian students because they offer the kind of supportive community in which gay and lesbian students can feel greater freedom to be themselves and not hide their sexual orientation.

? Are there college scholarships for gay students?

Yes, and they are generally for high school seniors who are headed to college. (You can find information about many of these scholarships through FinAid, a Web site that provides a "comprehensive annotated collection of information about student financial aid": www.finaid.org. Be sure to go to the section specifically devoted to financial aid for gay and lesbian students.)

One of the better-known scholarship funds is administered by the Point Foundation, which describes itself as "the first and only nationwide LGBT scholarship organization that focuses exclusively on granting assistance to undergraduate, graduate and post-graduate students of distinction." To get more information, you can visit the Point Foundation's Web site (www.thepointfoundation.org).

? Are there libraries and archives that specialize in gay subjects?

Several libraries around the country, including the San Francisco Public Library, the New York Public Library, and several university libraries, have—or are in the process of building—substantial gay and lesbian collections.

16

Politics and Activism

? Is homosexuality against the law?

No. It is not against the law to be a gay or lesbian person. There are no laws against feelings of sexual attraction. And there are no laws forbidding sexual relations between consenting adults of the same gender or opposite gender. But this has not always been the case.

Until 1961, all states had laws prohibiting sodomy, which made it illegal for adults to "perform or submit to any sexual act involving the sex organs of one person and the mouth or anus of another." Though these laws were rarely enforced, when they were, it was almost exclusively in cases involving sex between two men. (If these laws had been uniformly and aggressively enforced, one wonders how the jails would have accommodated everyone guilty of breaking these archaic rules.)

Beginning in 1961, through legislation or court action, state sodomy laws were eliminated in more than half the states. Then, in 2003, a U.S. Supreme Court decision in the case of *Lawrence v. Texas* eliminated the rest. The 2003 ruling reversed a 1986 Supreme Court decision that had upheld the state of

Georgia's sodomy laws in *Bowers v. Hardwick.* Both cases involved gay men who had been arrested in their own homes while engaging in consensual sexual relations.

? Why do gay and lesbian people feel they need laws to protect them from discrimination?

Given how much the world has changed in recent years for gay and lesbian people, it may be difficult to imagine what all the fuss is about and why gay people feel they need to be protected from discrimination through legislation at the federal, state, and local levels.

There's no question that things have changed dramatically since the 1950s, when gay people were routinely arrested and harassed by the police, fired from their jobs, expelled from universities, and denied housing. But if you pay attention to contemporary newspaper headlines, you'll see that gay people still face challenges in areas of their everyday lives that heterosexuals don't, including adoption and custody battles ("Court Rejects Visiting Rights for Former Lesbian Partner"), workplace discrimination ("Discriminating Against Gay Workers Doesn't Violate a U.S. Law), antigay violence ("Texas Judge Eases Sentence for Killer of 2 Homosexuals"), harassment ("Arkansas School Is Accused of Harassing a Gay Student"), and run-of-the-mill religious persecution ("Clerics of Three Faiths Protest Gay Festival Planned for Jerusalem").

The good news is that gay and lesbian people are protected by laws that forbid discrimination in employment, housing, and public accommodation in an ever-increasing number of states and municipalities. (The first city to pass gay rights legislation was Ann Arbor, Michigan, in July 1972).

Federal employees are also protected against discrimination. And a growing number of individual corporations, universities, and other public institutions have also adopted policies forbidding discrimination against gay and lesbian people in hiring and promotions.

For current information on states and municipalities that have antidiscrimination laws, visit the Web site for Lambda Legal (www.lambdalegal.org).

? What are the arguments against giving gay and lesbian people equal rights?

People who oppose the passage of gay and lesbian equal-rights laws and/or support their repeal give all kinds of reasons for their beliefs. Some argue that gay men and women are not a class of people—like those who are classified by race or gender—but simply individuals who engage in sick and sinful behavior that should not be protected by law.

I remember attending hearings at city hall in New York City during the early 1980s for local gay rights legislation, and I was more than a little disturbed by what I heard. One city councilman claimed that if gay people were given equal rights, the city would be encouraging bestiality and child molestation. (The bestiality argument—coupled with polygamy—is used to this day in the ongoing debate about granting gay people the legal right to marry.)

Seated in the row behind me in the second-floor balcony was a group of devoutly religious Jewish men—I am Jewish but not observant—who shouted "Burn them!" every time a gay person or supporter came up to the podium to testify. I thought these men, many of whom carried copies of the Bible and in all likelihood had relatives who had died in Hitler's gas chambers, made a very compelling case in *favor* of passing equal-rights protections for gay people. They also made me all the more grateful for the separation between church and state that is enshrined in thc U.S. Constitution.

Some antigay activists claim that gay people want "special rights," which is simply a lie. Gay and lesbian people are asking for the *same* legal protections most Americans take for granted, including protection from discrimination in employment, housing, and public accommodation. These are not "special rights." They are equal rights.

? Why are gay people fighting for the legal right to marry?

See chapter 6, "Dating, Relationships, and Marriage," for questions on this topic.

? When did the gay civil rights movement get its start?

The effort to free gay people from oppression and achieve equal rights began in California in the 1950s with the founding of two key organizations: the Mattachine Society, which was founded in Los Angeles by eight men in 1950; and the Daughters of Bilitis, an organization for lesbians founded in 1955.

These fledging groups had very modest goals that were a reflection of their tiny memberships, their modest resources, the intensely antigay climate of the times, and the overwhelming fear almost all gay and lesbian people had of being found out—which during that era could easily cost you your job.

Other than providing discussion groups where gay and lesbian people could meet one another and talk about the problems they faced, these organization fought for the right of gay people to assemble in bars without being harassed or arrested by the police, and they published the first widely circulated magazines for gay and lesbian people.

? Wasn't the 1969 Stonewall riot in New York City the beginning of the gay rights movement?

When I first began work on *Making Gay History,* my book about the gay and lesbian civil rights movement, I thought, like most other gay people, that the history of our struggle for equality began in 1969 with a June 28 riot that followed a routine police raid at the Stonewall Inn, a gay bar in New York City's Greenwich Village.

Well, I was off by nineteen years. Soon after I started my research and began interviewing gay rights pioneers, I discovered that by the time of the Stonewall riot there was already an active national movement of more than forty gay and lesbian organizations.

Although the Stonewall riot was not the beginning, it was, without question, a major turning point and very quickly became a symbol of gay people fighting back against oppression. It dramatically energized the movement and inspired the formation of scores of new, more radical, highly vocal and aggressive gay and lesbian rights groups across the country.

? Why do gay people have marches every year in June?

The annual gay and lesbian marches and celebrations commemorate the June 28, 1969, Stonewall riot in New York City.

These events are held in cities across the United States and in countries around the world, generally during the month of June.

Each local march or celebration committee sets its own theme, which may range from gay and lesbian freedom to gay pride. Each of the thousands of individual groups that appear in these local events has its own reasons for participating. And the hundreds of thousands of people who take part in the parades and celebrations have their own reasons as well.

Some people participate as a show of political strength, to celebrate gay and lesbian pride, to demand equal rights, or all of the above. Other people participate to express support for their gay and lesbian children or parents, or to celebrate the joy of not having to hide the truth about their lives. Still others are there just to have a good time.

One young woman I spoke with, who has been a regular participant in New York City's gay pride parade, gave this reason for marching: "It's the one day a year I can walk down the street in broad daylight with my arm around my girlfriend's shoulder and get cheered for it instead of having people spit at us."

Today's gay and lesbian marches and celebrations are a direct descendent of an annual protest march first held on July 4, 1965, in front of Independence Hall in Philadelphia. The protest was staged by a couple of dozen very courageous lesbians and gay men who carried signs demanding equal rights for homosexuals.

Martha Shelley, a gay rights leader in the late 1960s and early 1970s, participated in the Independence Hall protest two years in a row. "I thought it was something that might possibly have an effect," she recalled. "I remember walking around in my little white blouse and skirt, and tourists standing there eating their ice-cream cones and watching us like the zoo had opened."

Though virtually all Americans have now seen gay and lesbian people on television, in newspaper and magazine photographs, and in person, when the Independence Hall protests began, most people had never seen anyone who they knew was a living, breathing homosexual.

The Independence Hall annual protest continued through 1969. The following year, the Independence Hall protest was discontinued. Instead, a few thousand protesters marched in New York City on June 28 to commemorate the Stonewall riot, celebrate gay pride, and demand equal rights. Over a thousand protesters also marched that same day in Los Angeles.

? Why do gay people speak about gay pride? Straight people don't talk about heterosexual pride, do they?

I've always thought this question, with its follow-up kicker, was a little snotty. Of course straight people don't talk about heterosexual pride, because heterosexuality is embraced, celebrated, and "forced down our throats" just about every minute of every day. Where would the advertising industry be without heterosexual sex to help it sell everything from cars to carpeting?

In a more low-key way, heterosexual people express pride in their sexual orientation, whether they realize it or not, by having weddings, wearing wedding rings, and placing marriage announcements in newspapers. They're taking pride in their relationships, and I don't think there's anything wrong with that.

Now back to gay people. I like how Ann Northrop, an activist who has spoken widely on gay and lesbian rights issues, answered this question when I posed it to her. She said, "Homosexuals are taught from preconsciousness to be ashamed of themselves and to hate themselves and to think that they are disgusting, aberrant, immoral human beings. So the achievement of any kind of self-esteem in a lesbian or gay person is an incredible victory against almost insurmountable odds in the society we live in.

"Those of us who have achieved any small measure of self-esteem celebrate and take pride in the extent to which we've been able to achieve it. When you've been given the exact opposite all your life, there is a need to achieve a sense of pride."

Does the gay rights movement have its own Rosa Parks?

Although there is only one Rosa Parks, the late Dr. Evelyn Hooker, a pioneering research psychologist, has been called by some people "the Rosa Parks of the gay rights movement."

Dr. Hooker, who was heterosexual, conducted a courageous study in the 1950s in which she compared the psychological profiles of thirty homosexual men with the psychological profiles of thirty heterosexual men.

Dr. Hooker's work was courageous for two reasons. First, no one had ever thought to question the long-held assumption that gay people were by nature mentally ill. Second, she did her work during an extremely conservative and antigay period of American history. Undertaking such a study could easily have cost Dr. Hooker her career, especially given the study's outcome.

Dr. Hooker concluded that there were no significant differences between the two groups. Her findings ultimately led to the removal of homosexuality from the American Psychiatric Association's list of mental illnesses in 1973. This change in classification was one of the most important steps in the struggle for gay and lesbian equal rights, freeing millions of gay Americans from the stigma of what turned out to be a false mental-illness label.

What kinds of political organizations do gay and lesbian people have?

There are all kinds of organizations dedicated to working for gay rights, from high school and college student groups and political action committees to legal organizations and political clubs.

Among the most prominent national groups are the Gay and Lesbian Alliance Against Defamation (GLAAD); the Gay, Lesbian and Straight Education Network (GLSEN); the Human Rights Campaign (HRC); Lambda Legal; the National Gay and Lesbian Task Force (NGLTF); and Parents, Families and Friends of Lesbians and Gays (PFLAG). (See the "Resources" section in the back of this book for additional organizations and contact information.)

Why do some gay and lesbian people wear a pink triangle patch or button?

During World War II, the Nazis used an inverted (point-down) pink triangle symbol to identify homosexuals in concentration camps. (Jews had to wear a yellow Star of David.)

During the 1970s, as more became known about the persecution and murder of thousands of homosexuals by the Nazis, gay and lesbian people began wearing the inverted pink triangle symbol to publicly identify themselves as homosexuals, as a symbol of pride, and as a way of commemorating those who died in Hitler's concentration camps.

Why do some gay people fly a rainbow flag and display the rainbow symbol on their cars? Why do some stores, bars, and restaurants display a rainbow flag symbol in their windows?

It seems like rainbows are everywhere. Not just flags flown from front porches and decals on bumpers and car windows, but rainbow necklaces, rings, T-shirt insignia, towels, coffee mugs—you name it.

It all started with the six-stripe rainbow flag, which was designed and fabricated in 1978 by San Franciscan Gilbert Baker. His simple, subtle, and colorful symbol of gay and lesbian pride has been adopted around the world.

In the neighborhood where my partner and I live, the rainbow flag and rainbow decals are displayed in store windows to let gay and lesbian customers know that their patronage is more than welcome.

Are all lesbians and gay men liberals?

The vast majority of visible and politically active gay and lesbian people are comparatively liberal, so there is the mistaken impression that all gay people are Democrats and support liberal causes. But plenty of gay and lesbian people identify themselves as Republicans—including at least one U.S. congressman—and more than a few gay men and women are conservatives, including the late Marvin Liebman, who was a founder of the modern conservative movement. (The national organization for gay Republicans is called Log Cabin Republicans: www.logcabin.org.)

Some gay people have even been known to support and vote for conservative antigay candidates and to write antigay editorials. Don't ask me to explain this, because I can't.

? Is it true that the FBI once kept files on homosexuals?

From the 1950s through the early 1970s, gay and lesbian rights leaders claimed that the FBI was keeping a close eye on their activities. Some people thought that this was simply paranoia. It was *not* paranoia.

According to the late Randy Shilts, a journalist and the author of a best-selling book on the AIDS crisis, "The FBI conducted exhaustive and apparently illegal surveillance of the gay rights movement and its leaders for more than two decades.

"The surveillance started in 1953 and was continuing as late as 1975. Agents made extensive use of informants, tape-recorded meetings, collected lists of members of gay organizations, photographed participants in early homosexual rights marches, and investigated advertisers in gay publications."

17

Aging

? Are there gay and lesbian old people?

Yes, and my nephews think I'm one of them! But the truth is I'm just middle-aged.

When I first found my way into the gay world in New York City in the mid-1970s, my impression was that "old" gay people were around twenty-five or thirty. I rarely saw anyone much older, and I certainly never saw anyone over the age of fifty.

Where were all the older gay and lesbian people? For one thing, they weren't at the bars and clubs where I was going when I was in my late teens. And for that matter, you're not going to find older heterosexual people at the bars and clubs either.

Gay and lesbian older people tend to go on about their lives like all older people, and you're not likely to be able to tell them apart from heterosexual older people unless they're living as couples. And even then, plenty of older couples remain fairly private about the nature of their relationships, which is hardly surprising given the world in which they grew up.

For gay people now in their seventies and eighties, the world in which they came of age was one in which gay people were almost uniformly condemned and in which being open about your homosexuality was both unimaginable and dangerous. Is it any surprise, then, that many, if not most, remain cautious about the degree to which they're open about their lives?

In recent years, as gay men and lesbians of all ages have felt more comfortable with being open, increasing numbers of older gay men and women have made themselves known to their friends, families, and neighbors. And plenty of gay people who were once young activists, as well as those who have simply been accustomed to living openly and being treated equally, are reaching their fifties and sixties and will, no doubt, put a very visible face on what it means to be gay and gray.

? Are there old gay and lesbian couples?

Yes, and for my book about happy, long-lasting gay and lesbian relationships, I had the privilege of interviewing several older couples, including two women in their eighties who celebrated their fiftieth anniversary in 1998 and two men in their seventies who began their relationship shortly after the end of World War II.

? Is it harder growing old if you're gay or lesbian?

My grandmother would tell you that getting old is no picnic—for anyone. And that goes for gay people, too, although many older gay and lesbian people are more isolated than their heterosexual counterparts. Many, if not most, spent their lives hiding their sexual orientation and their relationships, and plenty plan to take their secret to the grave despite the changes in attitudes in recent decades.

Two older gay and lesbian people I've gotten to know over the years, Paul and Lena, have shared their secret with only a handful of gay friends, most of whom are now dead. Paul, who is nearly ninety, would like to let the people in his church know he's gay, but he's afraid they'll think less of him if they know the truth. "I've known I was homosexual since my teens, but I've always felt bad about it," said Paul, who lives by himself in an apartment complex for senior citizens in Denver. "I'd like to say something, but what if they don't accept me? What will I do then?"

Paul told me that he would like to find a companion, "not for a physical relationship—I can't do that anymore—but for the company." He asked me, "Do you think it's too late for me to meet someone?"

Lena, who is nearly eighty, lives in a small bungalow just outside Seattle with her two dogs and four cats. Only the two "gay boys" who live across the street from her know that she's a lesbian. "I think they knew I was gay soon after they moved in. I still haven't asked them how they could tell. We've gotten friendly over the past few years, and now we always share articles and books that talk about gays. Last week they drove me to the vet. One of the dogs was sick. I'm lucky to have them. They tell me they're lucky to have me."

For some gay and lesbian people, the sense of isolation can be extreme. They may have shared their secret with only one person—a long-term partner, for example. After the death of that partner, these men and women have no one with whom to share their lives and reminiscences and no one with whom they can be completely honest.

But isolation, though common, isn't everyone's experience. The two half-century couples I interviewed when I was working on my long-term-couples book are very visible in their respective communities in Delaware and Florida. While you're not likely to find them holding hands on the street, both couples make no effort to hide their relationships.

Shortly before I met the two women from Delaware, they were featured in their local newspaper. And the two men from Florida were called onstage during a public commitment ceremony for two hundred gay and lesbian couples at their church. When introduced to the assembled crowd, they were greeted with enthusiastic cheers.

Old age means all kinds of challenges for all men and women, but for gay people there's the added challenge of dealing with social-service agencies and health-care providers that may have no experience with gay men and lesbians. This can be especially difficult for couples who may be reluctant to reveal the relationship they have with their "best friend" or "housemate."

Imagine, for example, the challenge faced by a woman who needs to find a nursing home for her long-term partner who is suffering from severe memory loss, but doesn't want to reveal that they are more than just roommates. Because she and her beloved are just close friends—as far as the nursing home knows and in the eyes of the law—they will be treated very differently from a heterosexual married couple. And unless she and her partner have completed the necessary legal documents, the healthy partner will not be able to make medical and financial decisions for her ill spouse. Is it any wonder that gay people are fighting for the legal right to marry?

Are there organizations for older gay and lesbian people?

There are organizations for gay and lesbian senior citizens in most major cities. The oldest and best-known organization, SAGE—Senior Action in a Gay Environment—is located in New York City. SAGE is engaged in a range of efforts, from educating the public regarding the existence of gay elderly people to providing a range of services directly to elderly gay men and lesbians, primarily in New York City. SAGE also acts as a go-between for clients and government agencies, landlords, and hospitals. And it helps people find retirement homes that welcome gay and lesbian people. Visit the SAGE Web site (www.sageusa.org) for more information.

Are there gay retirement communities or nursing homes?

Some of my gay friends who have second homes in Palm Springs joke that Palm Springs is one big gay retirement home. In fact, there are several nursing homes and retirement communities geared specifically to gay people that are up and running or in development.

In addition, many care providers are beginning to address the fact that not all older people are straight. One social worker I spoke with, who works with nursing homes to make them aware of the special needs of gay and lesbian residents, told me that most nursing homes have a long way to go before they deal realistically with the issue of homosexuality.

What do grandchildren think of their gay grandparents?

In general, grandchildren are simply happy to have a loving grandparent and don't much care about sexual orientation one way or the other (although the parents might be an entirely different story).

One of my favorite stories on this topic comes from an interview in the *New York Times* several years ago. A seventy-nine-year-old woman, who asked to be identified as Gerry, said that when she told her daughter about her secret life, her daughter told her grandchildren, "Grandma's gay." According to the interview, "Gerry said that the kids looked at their mother and remarked, 'So what else is new?' Gerry smiled and said, 'It made me feel like I was only seventy years old.' "

Do gay people take care of elderly parents?

I've participated in more than a few discussions with gay friends where we've joked, sometimes ruefully, that God created gay people so we could take care of our elderly parents (while our siblings are busy raising their children). Although there are no statistics to back me up, anecdotally I know plenty of gay men and women who have stepped forward to care for an elderly relative.

My friends Jim and Lane, who live in rural North Carolina, are just one example. The two men took care of Lane's elderly mother for the last dozen years of her life. Lane told me, "She's got all these children—I'm one of nine—and nobody else would help her."

Jim and Lane did everything for Lane's mother, from helping her bathe to getting her to the doctor and watching over her medications. When her memory began to fail and she couldn't be left at home alone, they began taking her with them to work. Jim and Lane run a carpet cleaning and dyeing business.

Jim told me, "We couldn't get anyone to stay with her, and we didn't have the money to pay for anybody to stay with her. You do what you have to do when you ain't got the money to do it. So we had a van, which Lane remodeled. He put in captain's chairs, and he put a window in the side and installed an RV bathroom. Every morning we'd walk Mom up the ramp into the back of the van, and she'd go to Charlotte with us to clean carpets.

"We brought along our dog and our cat, and the cat would sit on Mom's lap all day. We did that for about two years, and Mom loved it. She had her picture window right by her seat, and she'd watch everything going on. And a lot of people at the apartment complexes got to know her, and they'd come and visit with her out at the truck. When the weather was pretty, we'd bring a lawn chair with us, and when we were doing a job, we'd put the lawn chair out and let Mom sit in the yard. She liked the routine, and it got her out of the house."

18

Miscellaneous Questions

? How do countries around the world deal with gay and lesbian people?

The range is pretty astonishing—from the Netherlands, where gay people have all the same rights as other Dutch citizens, including the legal right to marry, to countries where Islamic law is the law of the land and homosexual acts are illegal for both men and women and are punishable by death.

In general, gay people in most Western countries—including Canada and the member countries of the European Union—are protected by equal-rights laws. (The United States, which was at one time a leader in the realm of gay rights, now lags behind other Western countries.) Even in Russia, where sodomy laws were used from the 1930s until 1993 to send gay men to Siberian work camps, gay men and woman are now free from official sanctions, although they remain a generally scorned minority.

In other areas of the world, particularly parts of Asia and Africa, gay and lesbian people can face enormous oppression and may even fear for their lives. There are, of course, exceptions. For example, South Africa's constitution bans "unfair discrimination on the basis of sexual orientation," and in 2002 that nation's highest court ruled that laws forbidding adoptions by gay people were unconstitutional.

Many countries have no laws that forbid homosexual relations, but that doesn't mean gay and lesbian people in those countries can lead their lives in a climate free from prejudice or harm. In China, for example, gay people are sometimes treated for what most doctors there still consider a mental illness.

According to an article published in the *New York Times,* two of the most popular methods used in China to "cure" homosexuality are meant to discourage erotic thoughts, one through the application of painful electric shocks and the other through induced vomiting. On a brighter note, the article goes on to say that although most Chinese frown on homosexuality, it is considered in poor taste or improper rather than sinful. There are, the article adds, also "no common insults in Chinese related to sexual orientation."

Over the years, I've corresponded regularly with gay people from various countries around the world, including China, Jordan, Bangladesh, and Nepal. I wish I could say that what I've heard is news of sweeping and positive changes for gay people in these countries. But however difficult the lives are that they describe, what I find inspiring and hopeful is that the gay people I hear from yearn to live their lives like everyone else and are doing what they can within the limitations of their societies to meet other people like themselves, find relationships, and, when possible, organize for change.

For more information on gay rights around the world, visit the Web site for the International Gay and Lesbian Human Rights Commission (www.iglhrc.org).

? Why are there so many gay people in the United States? Are there as many gay people in other countries as there are in the United States?

This question came to me from a gay Vietnamese immigrant teenager. During a conversation one night at dinner, she heard a friend of her father's ask, "Why are there so many gay people here? Back in Vietnam we don't have gay people. We don't even have a name for them."

As the writer pointed out in her e-mail to me, there is indeed a word in Vietnamese for homosexuality. But because different cultures around the world have different attitudes toward homosexuality, it may appear in some countries that there are few or no homosexuals. This is especially true in countries where engaging in homosexual sex can land you in jail or cost you your life (though this is not the case in Vietnam).

The fact remains that across cultures and around the world, approximately the same percentage of the population has same-gender sexual orientation. The primary difference is how people choose to express—or not express—these feelings, most often in response to how different governments and cultures choose to deal with their gay and lesbian citizens.

In the United States, where the gay civil rights movement began in 1950, attitudes and laws are such that more gay people feel comfortable living their lives openly than in countries where homosexuality remains a taboo subject and gay rights efforts have yet to take hold.

? Can gay and lesbian people from countries outside the United States become U.S. citizens?

Until 1990, federal law barred people "with psychopathic personality, or sexual deviation, or a mental defect" from even entering the United States. This law was used to bar entry of homosexual aliens, and it was upheld in 1967, when the U.S. Supreme Court ruled that homosexuals could be barred from the country as sexual deviants.

In November 1990, the first President George Bush signed into law an immigration-reform bill that included the elimination of restrictions based on sexual orientation.

? Why do some gay men and lesbians dress up in black leather?

Sometimes gay and lesbian people, just like heterosexual people, wear black leather garments—pants, jackets, boots, and so on—simply because they like to wear black leather. It may be nothing more than a fashion statement.

For a relatively small number of gay men—and a smaller number of lesbians—black leather garments and accessories are an indication that they engage in S&M (sadism and masochism) role-playing and/or sex. Their black leather garments are part of a uniform that is recognized by other people who are a part of the "leather community." However, not all people who engage in S&M dress in black leather. And before you jump to any conclusions about S&M and gay people, please note that heterosexual people engage in such behavior as well.

? What is a transvestite? Are all transvestites gay men? Is that the same thing as a drag queen? And what is a drag king?

People use the words *transvestite* and *drag queen* to mean all kinds of different things, whether it's in reference to a gay man who likes to dress up in women's clothing for weekend parties or someone who dresses up in women's clothing and performs onstage. But the following are my official definitions based on my research.

A transvestite is someone who dresses in the clothing of the opposite sex and for whom that dressing is sexually exciting. Most transvestites are heterosexual men, and they do their cross-dressing in secret or only in the company of other heterosexual transvestites.

People who dress up in clothing of the opposite gender for a costume party, for a play, or just because they like doing it are said to be "cross-dressing" or dressing in "drag." A gay man who does this is sometimes called a *drag queen.* A lesbian who does this is sometimes called a *drag king.*

A man who dresses as a woman to perform professionally in public is called a *female impersonator.* But there are exceptions, such as Dame Edna (a.k.a., Barry Humphries). As everyone who has seen Dame Edna knows, Dame Edna is not Barry Humphries in drag. Dame Edna is simply, as she so modestly claims, a "giga-star."

? What is a drag show?

A drag show is just what it sounds like. It's a show—whether it takes place at a gay bar or on a theater stage—that features female impersonators. Typically the show involves impersonating a famous actress or performer, or inventing an entirely fictional character. There's usually lots of makeup, big hair, very high heels, and sequins. The performance can range from a comedy stand-up routine or lip-synching a variety of songs to doing a full-length one-"woman" show based on a fictional character or celebrity (living or dead).

? What is a drag ball?

One type of drag ball was featured in an acclaimed 1991 documentary by Jennie Livingston called *Paris Is Burning.* The film introduces viewers to Harlem drag balls, where African-American and Hispanic gay men and women dress up to compete for trophies in different categories. In the "Realness" category, for example, gay men try to "pass" as heterosexual schoolboys, executives, street thugs, soldiers, and beautiful, glamorous women.

Another type of drag ball is held in the context of the Imperial Court System, which is one of the oldest and largest gay charitable organizations in the United States. Dating back to the early 1960s, the several dozen individual "courts" of the Imperial Court System around the country hold fund-raising balls to benefit both local and national gay, as well as nongay, charities.

? Are gay men more sensitive than straight guys?

This is one of my favorite stereotypes! It certainly beats the stereotype that we're all child molesters.

Some gay men are indeed sensitive and understanding. And so are some straight men. But are gay men by nature more sensitive and understanding?

One theory I've heard over the years is that gay men are in general more sensitive than straight men because of their experience of growing up as an outsider. Because these men have to examine their lives and come to terms with something that makes them different from other men, they have more insight about life. This make them more sensitive than the average heterosexual man to the challenges faced by other people.

It's a nice theory, and I think it may even have some merit for some men, but one could also argue the opposite—that gay men are embittered by their experiences of growing up in a society hostile to gay people.

I don't think you have to choose one theory or another. Suffice it to say that there are gay men who are wonderfully sensitive and understanding, and there are others who are total blockheads. But on average, most gay men are just regular people.

? Why are gay men fans of opera?

Well, we can't seem to get away from stereotypes, but it does seem that there are a disproportionate number of gay men who can't resist the call of opera.

To me, opera's appeal is something of a mystery, because I can't get through *La Bohème* without falling asleep during the third act. And with Janáček's *Katia Kabanova,* I couldn't make it through the first act, despite the fact that I flew to Chicago to hear a friend who was singing a leading role. Fortunately my friend didn't glance down into the front row—she had gotten us house seats—to see me with my head slumped over, drooling on myself.

But I'm exaggerating (a little). I've really enjoyed seeing

Madame Butterfly and loved *Patience and Sarah,* a lesbian opera that premiered in 1998 at the Lincoln Center Summer Festival in New York City.

I asked one of my oldest friends, who has been an opera aficionado since college—though, he would say, not a true "opera queen"—what he thought the attraction was for gay men. He told me, "Opera aficionados can be of any gender or orientation. These are people who feel a deep connection with the drama, the music, and the spectacle.

"Opera queens," he said, "are focused on opera divas. They're there for the lead female singer. They are not interested in what else occurs on the stage, except perhaps for the rare attractive tenor over five feet tall. What they love about the divas is their combination of strength and vulnerability, but the crux of the opera queen's obsession is that the diva is bigger than life. They are watching someone act out, on a ridiculously vast scale, emotions that they can't begin to imagine acting out in their own lives."

My friend went on to note that "the classic opera queen is becoming less of a type as more men are able to lead openly gay lives. In the 1950s and '60s opera queens were typically men who had relatively dull lives and were uniformly closeted. Then in the dark of the theater they could completely fantasize and thrill to the fabulous icon of the opera diva. This sounds terrible to say, almost homophobic, but I think it was largely true of earlier generations of gay men who were forced to live such circumscribed lives. Opera gave them the opportunity to escape, and that's still one of the reasons all kinds of people enjoy opera."

My opera friend pointed out that there's even a subcategory of opera queens who are "high-note queens." These are gay men, he explained, who live solely for the auditory thrill of high notes produced by divas, whom they worship for their ability to sing these notes or denigrate for their failure to reach the musical stratosphere on key.

If you would like a book-length answer to the questions of why so many gay men love opera and what makes an "opera queen," I recommend reading *The Queen's Throat: Opera, Homosexuality, and the Mystery of Desire,* by Wayne Koestenbaum.

? Do all lesbians own Subarus?

Enough of the stereotypes! It just so happens, though, that a lot of lesbians do own Subarus (and so do my partner and I, which my gay sister-in-law jokes makes us honorary lesbians).

Subaru has taken note of their brand's popularity among lesbians and has made a concerted effort to reach the gay market through advertising.

? Do gay people have an impact on popular culture?

Gay and lesbian people have long had a major influence on popular culture, from the clothes people wear and the advertisements we see to the kind of music we dance to and the stories we read.

I like what the writer Fran Lebowitz has said on this subject: "If you removed all the homosexuals and homosexual influence from what is generally regarded as American culture, you would be pretty much left with *Let's Make a Deal.*" (*Let's Make a Deal* was a popular 1960s and 1970s television game show that featured contestants who dressed up in sometimes outlandish, and almost always embarrassing, costumes to compete for prizes.)

Bibliography

Aarons, Leroy. *Prayers for Bobby: A Mother's Coming to Terms with the Suicide of Her Gay Son.* San Francisco: HarperSanFrancisco, 1996.

Abelove, Henry. *The Lesbian and Gay Studies Reader.* New York and London: Routledge, 1993.

The Alyson Almanac, 1997: The Gay and Lesbian Fact Book and Guide to the Internet. Boston: Alyson Publications, 1997.

Bagemihl, Bruce. *Biological Exuberance: Animal Homosexuality and Natural Diversity.* New York: St. Martin's Press, 1999.

Barrett, Martha Barron. *Invisible Lives: The Truth About Millions of Women-Loving Women.* New York: Harper Perennial, 1990.

Bérubé, Allan. *Coming Out Under Fire: The History of Gay Men and Women in World War Two.* New York: The Free Press, 2000.

Berzon, Betty. *Permanent Partners: Building Gay and Lesbian Relationships That Last.* New York: Plume, 1990.

———. *Positively Gay: New Approaches to Gay and Lesbian Life.* Berkeley, CA: Celestial Arts, 2001.

Blumenthal, Warren J. *Homophobia: How We All Pay the Price.* Boston: Beacon Press, 1992.

Bono, Chastity. *Family Outing: A Guide to the Coming-Out Process for Gays, Lesbians, and Their Families.* New York: Little, Brown, 1998.

Borhek, Mary V. *My Son Eric: A Mother Struggles to Accept Her Gay Son and Discovers Herself.* New York: Pilgrim Press, 1984.

———. *Coming Out to Parents: A Two-Way Survival Guide for Lesbians and Gay Men and Their Parents.* New York: Pilgrim Press, 1993.

Boswell, John. *Christianity, Social Tolerance, and Homosexuality: Gay People in Western Europe from the Beginning of the Christian Era to the Fourteenth Century.* Chicago: Univ. of Chicago Press, 1981.

Boykin, Keith. *Beyond the Down Low: Sex, Lies, and Denial in Black America.* New York: Carroll & Graf, 2005.

Bright, Susie. *Susie Sexpert's Lesbian Sex World.* Pittsburgh: Cleis Press, 1990.

Buxton, Amity Pierce. *The Other Side of the Closet: The Coming-Out Crisis for Straight Spouses and Families.* Rev. ed. New York: John Wiley, 1994.

Cahill, Sean. *Same Sex Marriage in the United States: Focus on the Facts.* Lanham, MD: Lexington Books, 2004.

Crompton, Louis. *Homosexuality and Civilization.* Cambridge, MA: Belknap Press, 2003.

Curry, Hayden, and Dennis Clifford. *A Legal Guide for Lesbian and Gay Couples.* Berkeley, CA: Nolo Press, 2004.

DeGeneres, Betty. *Love, Ellen: A Mother/Daughter Journey.* New York: Perennial, 2000.

D'Emilio, John. *Sexual Politics, Sexual Communities: The Making of a Homosexual Minority in the United States, 1940 – 1970.* Chicago: Univ. of Chicago Press, 1998.

Dew, Robb Forman. *The Family Heart: A Memoir of When Our Son Came Out.* New York: Ballantine, 1995.

Duberman, Martin, Martha Vicinus, and George Chauncey Jr. *Hidden from History: Reclaiming the Gay and Lesbian Past.* New York: Plume, 1990.

Eichberg, Rob. *Coming Out: An Act of Love.* New York: Plume, 1991.

Faderman, Lillian. *Odd Girls and Twilight Lovers: A History of Lesbian Life in Twentieth-Century America.* New York: Penguin, 1992.

———. *To Believe in Women: What Lesbians Have Done for America —A History.* Boston: Houghton Mifflin, 1999.

Fairchild, Betty, and Nancy Hayward. *Now That You Know: A Parents' Guide to Understanding Their Gay and Lesbian Children.* New York: Harcourt Brace Jovanovich, 1998.

Fricke, Aaron. *Reflections of a Rock Lobster: A Story About Growing Up Gay.* St. Paul: Consortium, 1995.

Garber, Marjorie. *Bisexuality and the Eroticism of Everyday Life.* New York and London: Routledge, 2000.

Gates, Gary J., and Jason Ost. *The Gay and Lesbian Atlas.* Washington DC: Urban Institute, 2004.

Griffin, Carolyn Welch, Marian J. Wirth, and Arthur G. Wirth. *Beyond Acceptance: Parents of Lesbians and Gays Talk About Their Experiences.* Englewood Cliffs, NJ: Prentice-Hall, 1986.

Harwood, Gean. *The Oldest Gay Couple in America: A Seventy-Year Journey Through Same-Sex America.* New York: Birch Lane Press, 1997.

Heger, Heinz. *The Men with the Pink Triangle.* Boston: Alyson Publications, 1980.

Helminiak, Daniel A. *What the Bible Really Says About Homosexuality.* Sacramento, CA: Alamo Square, 2000.

Herek, Gregory M. *Hate Crimes: Confronting Violence Against Lesbians and Gay Men.* Newbury Park, CA: Sage Publications, 1992.

Heron, Ann. *Two Teenagers in Twenty: Writings by Gay and Lesbian Youth.* Boston: Alyson Publications, 1995.

Hobson, Laura Z. *Consenting Adult.* New York: Warner Books, 1976.

Hunter, Nan D., Courtney G. Joslin, and Sharon M. McGowan. *The Rights of Lesbians, Gay Men, Bisexuals, and Transgender People: The Authoritative ACLU Guide to the Rights of Lesbians, Gay Men, Bisexuals, and Transgendered People.* 4th ed. American Civil Liberties Union Handbook. New York: NYU Press, 2004.

Hutchings, Loraine, and Lani Kaahumanu. *Bi Any Other Name: Bisexual People Speak Out.* Boston: Alyson Publications, 1991.

Isay, Richard A. *Being Homosexual: Gay Men and Their Development.* New York: Avon Books, 1989.

Jennings, Kevin, ed. *Becoming Visible: A Reader in Gay and Lesbian History for High School and College Students.* Boston: Alyson Publications, 1994.

———. *Always My Child: A Parent's Guide to Understanding Your Gay, Lesbian, Bisexual, Transgendered or Questioning Son or Daughter.* New York: Fireside, 2002.

Koestenbaum, Wayne. *The Queen's Throat: Opera, Homosexuality, and the Mystery of Desire.* Cambridge, MA: Da Capo Press, 2001.

Kopay, David, and Perry Deane Young. *The David Kopay Story.* New York: Bantam, 1977.

Marcus, Eric. *Making Gay History: The Half-Century Fight for Lesbian and Gay Equal Rights.* New York: HarperCollins, 2002.

———. *The Male Couple's Guide: Finding a Man, Making a Home, Building a Life.* New York: HarperCollins, 1999.

———. *Together Forever: Gay and Lesbian Couples Share Their Secrets for Lasting Happiness.* New York: Anchor, 1999.

———. *What If Someone I Know Is Gay? Answers to Questions About Gay and Lesbian People.* New York: Penguin Putnam/Price, Stern, Sloan, 2000.

Martin, April. *The Lesbian and Gay Parenting Handbook: Creating and Raising Our Families.* New York: HarperCollins, 1993.

McNaught, Brian. *Now That I'm Out, What Do I Do?* New York: St. Martin's Press, 1997.

McNeill, John J. *The Church and the Homosexual.* 4th ed. Boston: Beacon Press, 1993.

Miller, Neil. *In Search of Gay America: Women and Men in a Time of Change.* New York: HarperCollins, 1990.

———. *Out in the World: Gay and Lesbian Life from Buenos Aires to Bangkok.* New York: Random House, 1992.

Muller, Ann. *Parents Matter: Parents' Relationships with Lesbian Daughters and Gay Sons.* Tallahassee, FL: Naiad Press, 1987.

Pallone, Dave. *Behind the Mask: My Double Life in Baseball.* New York: Viking, 1990.

Pies, Cheri. *Considering Parenthood.* San Francisco: Spinsters, 1988.

Plant, Richard. *The Pink Triangle: The Nazi War Against Homosexuals.* New York: Henry Holt and Company, 1986.

Russo, Vito. *The Celluloid Closet: Homosexuality in the Movies.* New York: Perennial, 1987.

Schow, Ron, Wayne Schow, and Marybeth Raynes. *Peculiar People: Mormons and Same-Sex Orientation.* Salt Lake City: Signature Books, 1991.

Schulenburg, Joy A. *Gay Parenting: A Complete Guide for Gay Men and Lesbians with Children.* Garden City, NY: Anchor Press, 1985.

Sember, Brette McWhorter. *Gay and Lesbian Rights: A Guide for GLBT Singles, Couples and Families.* Naperville, IL: Sphinx, 2003.

Sherman, Suzanne. *Lesbian and Gay Marriage: Private Commitments, Public Ceremonies.* Philadelphia: Temple Univ. Press, 1992.

Shilts, Randy. *And the Band Played On: Politics, People, and the AIDS Epidemic.* New York: St. Martin's Press, 1987.

———. *Conduct Unbecoming: Gays and Lesbians in the U.S. Military.* New York: St. Martin's Press, 1993.

Signorile, Michelangelo. *Outing Yourself: How to Come Out as Lesbian or Gay to Your Family, Friends, and Coworkers.* New York: Fireside, 1996.

Spong, John Shelby. *Living in Sin? A Bishop Rethinks Human Sexuality.* San Francisco: HarperSanFrancisco, 1988.

Stevenson, Michael R, and Jeanine C. Cogan. *Everyday Activism: A Handbook for Lesbian, Gay, and Bisexual People and Their Allies.* New York: Routledge, 2003

Strah, David. *Gay Dads: A Celebration of Fatherhood.* New York: Tarcher, 2003.

Uhrig, Larry J. *The Two of Us: Affirming, Celebrating and Symbolizing Gay and Lesbian Relationships.* Boston: Alyson Publications, 1984.

Vacha, Keith. *Quiet Fire: Memoirs of Older Gay Men.* Trumansburg, NY: The Crossing Press, 1985.

Van Gelder, Lindsy, and Pamela Robin Brandt. *Are You Two . . . Together? A Gay and Lesbian Travel Guide to Europe.* New York: Random House, 1991.

Resources

HIV/AIDS and Sexually Transmitted Diseases

Centers for Disease Control 24-hour telephone hotlines
National STD Hotline: 800-227-8922
National AIDS Hotline: 800-342-AIDS

Centers for Disease Control
www.cdc.gov

National Center for HIV, STD and TB Prevention
www.cdc.gov/hiv/dhap.htm

Division of Sexually Transmitted Diseases
www.cdc.gov/std/

Organizations

Children of Lesbians and Gays Everywhere (COLAGE)
3543 18th Street, #1
San Francisco, CA 94110
415-861-KIDS (5437)
www.colage.org
collage@colage.org

The Commercial Closet
P.O. Box 20516
New York, NY 10009-9991
212-995-0147
www.commercialcloset.org

Family Pride Coalition
P.O. Box 65327
Washington, DC 20035-5327
202-331-5015
www.familypride.org
info@familypride.org

FinAid
10 St. Francis Way, #9-134
Cranberry Township, PA
16066-5126
724-538-4500
www.finaid.org
questions@finaid.org

Gay and Lesbian Advocates and Defenders (GLAD)
30 Winter Street, Suite 800
Boston, MA 02108
617-426-1350
www.glad.org

Gay and Lesbian Alliance Against Defamation (GLAAD)
248 West 35th Street,
8th Floor
New York, NY 10001
212-629-3322
www.glaad.org

Gay and Lesbian Victory Fund
1705 DeSales Street, NW,
#500
Washington, DC 20036
202-842-8679
www.victoryfund.org
victory@victoryfund.org

Gay, Lesbian and Straight Education Network (GLSEN)
121 West 27th Street, #804
New York, NY 10001
212-727-0135
www.glsen.org
glsen@glsen.org

Hetrick-Martin Institute
2 Astor Place
New York, NY 10003
212-674-2400
www.hmi.org
info@hmi.org

Human Rights Campaign
1640 Rhode Island
Avenue, NW
Washington, DC 20036-3278
202-628-4160
www.hrc.org
hrc@hrc.org

Human Rights Campaign
National Coming Out Project
www.hrc.org/comingout

International Gay and Lesbian Human Rights Commission
350 Fifth Avenue, 34th Floor
New York, NY 10118
212-216-1814
www.iglhrc.org
iglhrc@iglhrc.org

Lambda Legal
120 Wall Street, #15
New York, NY 10005
212-809-8585
www.lambdalegal.org
legalhelpdesk@lambdalegal.org

National Coalition of Anti-Violence Programs (NCAVP)
240 West 35th Street, #200
New York, NY 10001

212-714-1184
www.ncavp.org
info@ncavp.org

National Gay and Lesbian Task Force (NGLTF)
1325 Massachusetts Avenue, NW, #600
Washington, DC 20005
202-393-5177
www.thetaskforce.org
thetaskforce@thetaskforce.org

National Lesbian & Gay Journalists Association (NLGJA)
420 K Street, NW, #910
Washington, DC 20005
202-588-9888
www.nlgja.org
info@nlgja.org

National Youth Advocacy Coalition (NYAC)
1638 R Street, NW, #300
Washington, DC 20009
202-319-7596
800-541-6922 (toll-free)
www.nyacyouth.org
nyac@nyacyouth.org

Parents, Families and Friends of Lesbians and Gays (PFLAG)
1726 M Street, NW, #400
Washington, DC 20036
202-467-8180
www.pflag.org
info@pflag.org

Senior Action in a Gay Environment (SAGE)
305 7th Avenue, 16th Floor
New York, NY 10001
212-741-2247
www.sageusa.org

Servicemembers Legal Defense Network (SLDN)
P.O. Box 65301
Washington, DC 20035-5301
202-328-3244
www.sldn.org
sldn@sldn.org

Straight Spouse Network
8215 Terrace Drive
El Cerrito, CA 94530-3058
510-525-0200
www.ssnetwk.org

Index